International Congress and Symposium Series

Editor-in-Chief: Hugh L'Etang

The position of bopindolol

a new β-blocker

Proceedings of a Round Table Conference sponsored by Sandoz Cardiovasculars, The Netherlands (Uden) held in Amsterdam, 23 May 1986

International Congress and Symposium Series
Number 106

The position of bopindolol
a new β-blocker

Edited by
P. A. van Zwieten

Royal Society of Medicine Services
London New York
1987

Royal Society of Medicine Services Limited
1 Wimpole Street London W1M 8AE
7 East 60th Street New York NY 10022

These proceedings are published by Royal Society of Medicine Services Ltd with financial support from the sponsor. The contributors are responsible for the scientific content and for the views expressed, which are not necessarily those of the Royal Society of Medicine or of Royal Society of Medicine Services Ltd. Distribution has been in accordance with the wishes of the sponsor but a copy is available to any Fellow of the Society at a privileged price.

British Library Cataloguing in Publication Data
The position of bopindolol, a new beta-blocker.—
(International congress and symposium series; no. 106)
1. Bopindolol
I. Zwieten P. A. van II. Royal Society of Medicine
III. Series
615'.71 RM666.B6

ISBN 0-905958-36-5

Editorial and production services by Fisher Duncan Ltd, 10 Barley Mow Passage, London W4 4PH
Phototypeset by Dobbie Typesetting Service, Plymouth, Devon
Printed in Great Britain at the University Press, Oxford

Contributors

Editor

P. A. van Zwieten
Faculty of Medicine, Division of Pharmacotherapy, University of Amsterdam, Plantage Muidergracht 24, 1018 TV, Amsterdam, The Netherlands

O. K. Andersson
Department of Medicine I, Sahlgrenska Hospital, 413 45 Göteborg, Sweden

S. H. Braat
University Hospital of Maastricht, University of Limburg, PO Box 1918, 6201 BX Maastricht, The Netherlands

O.-E. Brodde
Biochemical Research Laboratories, Medical Clinic and Policlinic, Division of Renal and Hypertensive Diseases, University Hospital of Essen, D-4300 Essen, Federal Republic of Germany

P. van Brummelen
Department of Nephrology, University Hospital Leiden, PO Box 9600, 2300 RC Leiden, The Netherlands

F. R. Bühler
Department of Medicine, University Hospital, Basle, Switzerland

J.-C. Bousquet
Medical Policlinic, University of Bern, Freiburgstrasse 3, 3010 Bern, Switzerland

C. Christensen
Clinic for Cardiology and Medicine, St Olavs Plass 1, Oslo, Norway

A. J. M. Donker
Department of Medicine, Free University Hospital, De Boelelaan 1117, 1007 MB Amsterdam, The Netherlands

P. Fitscha
2nd Department of Internal Medicine (Heartstation), General Policlinic, Mariannengasse 10, A-1090 Vienna, Austria

O. Galal
Biochemical Research Laboratories, Medical Clinic and Policlinic, Division of Renal and Hypertensive Diseases, University Hospital of Essen, D-4300 Essen, Federal Republic of West Germany

A. P. M. Gorgels
University Hospital of Maastricht, University of Limburg, PO Box 1918, 6201 BX Maastricht, The Netherlands

J. Grevel
Department of Materia Medica, Stobhill General Hospital, University of Glasgow, Glasgow G21 3UW, United Kingdom

E. Hardy
University Hospital of Maastricht, University of Limburg, PO Box 1918, 6201 BX Maastricht, The Netherlands

T. Hedner
Department of Clinical Pharmacology, Sahlgrenska University Hospital, 41345 Göteborg, Sweden

A. J. Man in 't Veld
Department of Internal Medicine I, University Hospital Dijkzigt, Dr. Molewaterplein 40, 3015 GD Rotterdam, The Netherlands

A. H. van den Meiracker
Department of Internal Medicine I, University Hospital Dijkzigt, Dr. Molewaterplein 40, 3015 GD Rotterdam, The Netherlands

W. Meisner
2nd Department of Internal Medicine (Heartstation), General Policlinic, Mariannengasse 10, A-1090 Vienna, Austria

G. Nyberg
Department of Medicine, Östra Hospital, S-416 Göteborg, Sweden

M. A. D. H. Schalekamp
Department of Internal Medicine I, University Hospital Dijkzigt, Dr. Molewaterplein 40, 3015 GD Rotterdam, The Netherlands

B. Tiso
2nd Department of Internal Medicine (Heartstation), General Policlinic, Mariannengasse 10, A-1090, Vienna, Austria

A. Vermeulen
Andreas Hospital, Theophile de Bockstraat 8, 1058 NR Amsterdam, The Netherlands

X. L. Wang
Biochemical Research Laboratories, Medical Clinic and Policlinic, Division of Renal and Hypertensive Diseases, University Hospital of Essen, D-4300 Essen, Federal Republic of Germany

P. Weidmann
Medical Policlinic, University of Bern, Freiburgstrasse 3, 3010 Bern, Switzerland

R. F. Westerman
Department of Medicine, Free University Hospital, De Boelelaan 1117, 1007 MB Amsterdam, The Netherlands

A. Westheim
Clinic for Cardiology and Medicine, St Olavs Plass 1, Oslo, Norway

Contents

Preface

The management of essential hypertension with β-adrenoceptor blocking drugs has been widely applied and in the majority of cases satisfactory control without unacceptable side-effects is achieved. The number of compounds continues to increase, although at a slower pace than previously. β_1-Selectivity, intrinsic sympathomimetic activity (ISA) and duration of action are the most relevant ancillary properties of individual β-blockers. β-Blockers with several combinations of these ancillary properties have become available over the years. In the treatment of hypertension a once daily dosage of drug is recognized more and more as a useful property which improves compliance. For this reason the tendency to develop long-acting β-blockers, as antihypertensives and also in the long-term treatment of angina pectoris, is understandable. Bopindolol is an example of a potent and unusually long-acting β-adrenoceptor blocking agent. These properties of the new compound are not only interesting for theoretical reasons, but also potentially useful to the drug's application as an antihypertensive.

On 23 May, 1986, a Round Table Conference by experts in the field was devoted to the profile of bopindolol compared with that of established β-blockers. The most important aspects of the field were covered, included both fundamental and clinical aspects.

A fairly complete and up to date survey has been obtained, as can be seen from this publication. It is my pleasure as a chairman of the conference and as editor of the publication to acknowledge the gratitude of the participants to Sandoz-Nederland (Uden). The company provided generous hospitality, leaving the scientific responsibility, however, entirely to the chairman and speakers.

P. A. van Zwieten

Different properties of β-adrenoceptor blockers: characteristics of bopindolol

P. A. VAN ZWIETEN

Faculty of Medicine, Division of Pharmacotherapy, University of Amsterdam, Amsterdam, The Netherlands

Summary

A survey is given of the principle of β-adrenoceptor blockade and its sequelae. β_1-Adrenoceptor selectivity, intrinsic sympathomimetic activity (ISA) and membrane stabilization are ancillary properties of certain β-blockers. The basic aspects and relevance of these properties are explained. Furthermore, a survey is given of the most important therapeutic applications of β-adrenoceptor blockers, as well as the backgrounds of their side-effects, contraindications and interactions with other drugs. Finally, a brief characterization is given of the newly introduced β-adrenoceptor blocking agent bopindolol.

Introduction

In the adrenergic nervous system, noradrenaline is the dominant neurotransmitter, whereas adrenaline is, at least quantitatively, of lesser importance. The adrenoceptors in this system are divided into the α and β subtypes, according to the receptor demand of these receptor subtypes. α-Adrenoceptor subtypes are present at both pre- and postsynaptic locations. At presynaptic sites mainly α_2-adrenoceptors are found; postsynaptic α-adrenoceptors are known to comprise both α_1- and α_2-adrenoceptor subtypes. It should be emphasized that the terms α_1 and α_2 refer to the receptor demand, whereas the expressions pre- and postsynaptic reflect the position with respect to the synapse. Postsynaptic α_1- and α_2-adrenoceptors both induce vasoconstriction when stimulated by their respective agonists (1).

β-Adrenoceptors are also subdivided into pre- and postsynaptic subtypes. The excitation of presynaptic (prejunctional) β-adrenoceptors facilitates the release of endogenous noradrenaline, whereas their blockade inhibits the mobilization of

The position of bopindolol, a new β-blocker, edited by P. A. van Zwieten, 1987: Royal Society of Medicine Services International Congress and Symposium Series No. 106, published by Royal Society of Medicine Services Limited.

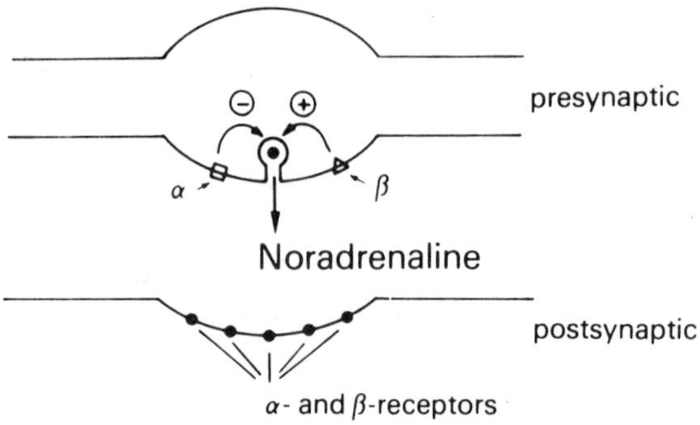

Figure 1. α- and β-Adrenoceptors at pre- and postsynaptic sites. The stimulation of presynaptic α-adrenoceptors inhibits the release of noradrenaline from the varicosity where it is stored. However, stimulation of presynaptic β-receptors enhances the release of the neurotransmitter from the nerve ending. Conversely, the blockade of presynaptic β-receptors diminishes the release of noradrenaline. Once noradrenaline has been released, it travels through the synaptic cleft and reaches both α- and β-adrenoceptors at postsynaptic sites, thus causing physiological effects such as vasoconstriction or tachycardia.

endogenous noradrenaline (Fig. 1). β-Adrenoceptors are located, for instance, in the heart, the bronchi, and the gut, whereas various biochemical processes like the liberation of glucose from glycogen are also known to be mediated by β-receptors. At present, β-receptors are divided into β_1 and β_2 subtypes (2,3). The postsynaptic β_1-adrenoceptors are involved mainly in the regulation of cardiac function. Their stimulation causes an increase in cardiac frequency and contractility. Excitation of β_2-adrenoceptors by the appropriate agonists induces bronchodilatation, vasodilatation, and hyperglycaemia. The classic β-adrenoceptor agonists, such as, for instance, isoprenaline and orciprenaline, are non-selective; i.e., they stimulate β_1- and β_2-adrenoceptors equally well. Presynaptic β-adrenoceptors mainly belong to the β_2-subtype.

Selective β_2-adrenoceptor stimulants such as terbutaline and salbutamol influence predominantly the bronchi without causing excessive tachycardia. For this reason they are preferred as bronchospasmolytic agents over the non-selective $\beta_1 + \beta_2$-adrenoceptor agonists (isoprenaline, orciprenaline), which are known to provoke substantial complaints of tachycardia and palpitations.

More recently, dobutamine has been introduced as a rather selective β_1- adrenoceptor agonist, but it also possesses significant α_1-agonistic potency (4).

β-Sympatholytic drugs, β-adrenoceptor blocking agents

The β-adrenoceptor blocking agents possess substantial affinity for the receptors, so that the receptors are blocked and thus become inaccessible to agonists such as the endogenous neurotransmitters or the aforementioned synthetic β-sympathomimetic receptor agonists. The β-receptor agonists combine with the receptor, so that the drug-receptor complex is formed, without giving rise to receptor activation as observed for an agonistic compound (2).

The inaccessibility of the receptor for endogenous catecholamines (noradrenaline, adrenaline) considerably diminishes or even abolishes the influence of the sympathetic nervous system on various organs, although the sympathetic fibres are entirely intact.

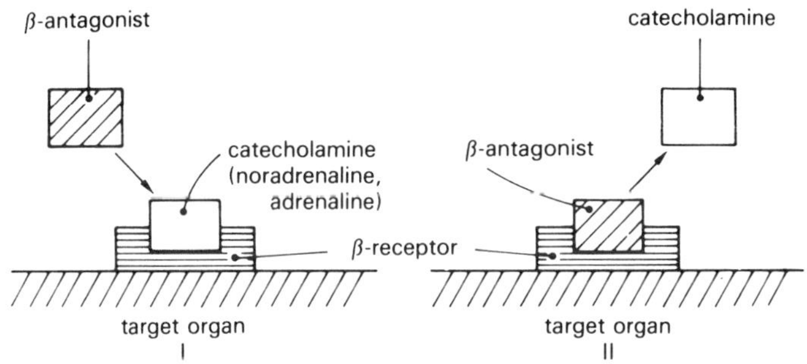

Figure 2. Principle of competitive antagonism at the level of β-adrenoceptors. An endogenous catecholamine (noradrenaline, adrenaline) combines with the receptor and causes a stimulus, leading to a physiological or pharmacological effect (e.g. tachycardia). A β-adrenoceptor blocking agent combines with the receptor without causing a stimulus. However, the receptor is blocked and therefore no longer accessible to endogenous catecholamines or external synthetic β-adrenoceptor agonists.

Competition exists between the neurotransmitter and the β-blocking agent for the β-adrenoceptor, thus justifying the application of the term competitive antagonism for the given situation (Fig. 2).

Various properties of β-adrenoceptor blocking agents

All therapeutically applied β-adrenoceptor blocking agents are known to block β_1-adrenoceptors. Most therapeutic effects, but not all, are based on β_1-adrenoceptor blockade (see below). Various β-blockers are known to substantially block β_2-adrenoceptors as well. This is particularly the case for the so-called non-selective β-blockers. In most cases the β_2-adrenoceptor blockade causes side-effects. Only in a few cases, i.e., in the treatment of glaucoma and in certain forms of tremor, is β_2-blockade known to be the basis of the therapeutic effect. Bronchoconstriction and vasoconstriction are known to be induced by β_2-receptor blockade (2).

Apart from the blocking activity of β-sympatholytic agents, various compounds in this series possess other properties, such as membrane-stabilizing (local anaesthetic) potency and/or intrinsic sympathomimetic activity (ISA). These properties shall be dealt with separately below, together with the so-called cardioselectivity of β-adrenoceptor blocking agents, which is based on the preferential antagonistic activity of certain β-blockers for β_1-adrenoceptors.

Cardioselectivity of β-blockers

Since in the cardiovascular field all therapeutic effects of β-blockers are based on β_1-receptor blockade, whereas in most cases the blockade of β_2-receptors causes unpleasant and sometimes dangerous side-effects, a great effort has been invested in the development of β-receptor blocking drugs with a preferential affinity toward β_1-receptors. Some compounds with such a preferential affinity have indeed been developed. So far, however, the selectivity of this type of drug has remained limited. Even when the expression β_1-receptor selectivity might be acceptable, the term cardioselectivity is certainly not justified for the compounds available at present (5).

In spite of a preferential affinity for β_1-adrenoceptors, the β-sympatholytic compounds classified as cardioselective still display so much affinity for β_2-adrenoceptors that they are certainly not safe in patients suffering from obstructive airways diseases like bronchial asthma. Moreover, the bronchi have been demonstrated to contain a limited density of β_1-adrenoceptors. It should be recognized, however, that the severity of the impairment of ventilation is certainly less than that observed for non-selective $\beta_1+\beta_2$-adrenoceptor blocking agents (5,6).

The expression cardioselective has been widely used; it would be preferable to classify the drugs involved as β_1-receptor selective. Well-known examples of rather selective β_1-adrenoceptor blocking agents (at least in low doses) are atenolol, metoprolol, practolol (virtually no more applied), and to a lesser degree acebutolol (see Table 1).

Table 1

Various β-adrenoceptor blocking agents and their differentiation with respect to membrane stabilization, β_1-selectivity, and intrinsic sympathomimetic activity (ISA).

Drug	β_1-selectivity	Membrane stabilization	ISA
Acebutolol	$\beta_1>\beta_2$	−	+
Alprenolol	$\beta_1+\beta_2$	±	+
Atenolol	$\beta_1>>\beta_2$	−	−
Betaxolol	$\beta_1>>\beta_2$	±	−
Bopindolol	$\beta_1+\beta_2$	−	+
Metoprolol	$\beta_1>>\beta_2$	−	−
Metipranolol	$\beta_1+\beta_2$	−	−
Oxprenolol	$\beta_1+\beta_2$	±	+ +
Penbutolol	$\beta_1+\beta_2$	±	+
Pindolol	$\beta_1+\beta_2$	−	+ + +
Practolol	$\beta_1>>\beta_2$	−	+ +
Propranolol	$\beta_1+\beta_2$	+	−
Sotalol	$\beta_1+\beta_2$	−	−
Timolol	$\beta_1+\beta_2$	−	−

$\beta_1+\beta_2$: non-selective compound; $\beta_1>>\beta_2$ β_1 selectivity.

Membrane stabilization (local anaesthetic activity)

Various β-adrenoceptor blocking agents are known to influence the cell membrane in an unspecific manner, besides the more or less specific blocking activity of the β-adrenoceptors. The direct effect on the cell membrane, classified as membrane-stabilizing, local anaesthetic, or quinidine-like activity, is known to reduce the membrane permeability for various ions, such as sodium, potassium, and calcium. These effects are unrelated to β-adrenoceptor blockade (7). Membrane stabilization as discussed above is very similar to local anaesthetic activity. As such it causes bradycardia and reduction of contractility and of the rate of atrioventricular (AV) conduction. Accordingly, the cardiac output is also reduced (8).

Membrane stabilization does not influence, in either the positive or negative sense, the therapeutic efficacy of β-receptor blockade. The drugs involved do not display substantial membrane-stabilizing activity. It has been argued that the membrane-stabilizing activity of β-blockers contributes to the antiarrhythmic potency of these drugs but this argument seems questionable (8).

Concerning the classical β-blocker propranolol it seems of interest to mention that both optical (stereo-)isomers of this compound display substantial and comparable membrane-stabilizing activity, whereas the β-adrenoceptor blocking potency remains limited to one of the two isomers, the other being devoid of such activity (2). Propranolol, alprenolol, and oxprenolol are well-known examples of β-blocking agents that possess membrane-stabilizing potency (see Table 1).

ISA

β-Adrenoceptor blocking agents will cause the formation of a drug-receptor complex with β-adrenoceptors; accordingly, all β-blockers are bound to possess affinity toward the β-receptor. Certain drugs, for instance, pindolol, oxprenolol, and alprenolol, not only display affinity toward the receptor, but also possess a mild degree of agonistic potency. Accordingly, the receptor is blocked and inaccessible to endogenous catecholamines (noradrenaline, adrenaline), whereas the β-blocker in question mildly stimulates the β-adrenoceptor. In molecular pharmacology, this phenomenon is characterized as partial agonism.

The various backgrounds of ISA have been dealt with in full detail by Ariëns (9). In Table 1 the various properties of currently available β-adrenoceptor blocking agents have been enumerated.

Therapeutic applications of β-adrenoceptor blocking agents

Cardiovascular disease

β-Adrenoceptor blocking agents have gained an important position as drugs of choice in the treatment of hypertension and angina pectoris. The treatment of tachyarrhythmia with β-blockers is a more refined and less generally applied application of these drugs. The antihypertensive potency of β-blockers has not as yet been satisfactorily explained. The following mechanisms have been put forward as a possible basis of the antihypertensive potency of β-blocking agents: reduction of cardiac output; a central mechanism; reduction of plasma renin activity; and blockade of presynaptic β_2-adrenoceptors (8,10). None of these mechanisms has proved to be satisfactory as an explanation of the antihypertensive effect of β-blocking agents. Neither is it possible to dismiss with certainty one or more of these mechanisms as being wholly incorrect. The antihypertensive effect of β-adrenoceptor blocking agents is based on the blockade of β_1-adrenoceptors. Cardioselectivity and membrane stabilization are of no consequence whatsoever with respect to the antihypertensive effect as such. Intrinsic sympathomimetic activity does not lead to a stronger or weaker antihypertensive effect. However, the haemodynamic profile of a β-blocker with ISA is different from that of a drug devoid of this property (11,12).

In the chronic treatment of classic exercise-induced angina pectoris with β-blocking agents, the reduced or abolished influence of endogenous catecholamines on the heart gives rise to a diminishment of myocardial oxygen consumption, thus improving the ratio of oxygen supply to demand, which is known to be disturbed in this disorder (13). In particular the reduction in cardiac frequency reduces oxygen consumption. β-Blockers are unsuitable for the interruption of an acute attack of angina, which should preferentially be treated with nitroglycerin or isosorbine dinitrate. Prinzmetal angina, which is assumed to be due to coronary spasm, is, as a rule, unfavourably influenced by β-adrenoceptor blocking agents. This rare type of angina should preferentially be treated with a calcium entry blocker, such as nifedipine (14).

The therapeutic effect of β-blockers in angina is probably based on β_1-adrenoceptor blockade only. Theoretically, all β-blockers developed so far would be useful as antianginal drugs, but not all of them have been studied systematically in this connection. No studies exist that would indicate that properties like β_1 selectivity, membrane stabilization, or ISA would be of particular benefit or disadvantage to the antianginal effect as such (13,15).

The antiarrhythmic effect of β-blockers in the usual doses is due only to their β-adrenoceptor blocking activity, because membrane stabilization occurs only at much higher doses. This indicates that β-adrenoceptor blocking agents can be applied in those conditions where enhanced sympathetic activity facilitates the occurrence of dysrhythmia, like anxiety, physical stress, general anaesthesia, and myocardial ischaemia. The rate of firing of the sinus node and also that of other cells in the heart showing spontaneous discharges is reduced by β-blockers. Therefore, atrial and ventricular dysrhythmias caused by abnormal automaticity can be treated with β-blockers. The increase in AV conduction time and the enhanced refractory period of the AV node by β-blockers explain the efficacy of these drugs in arrhythmias in which the AV node plays an important part (16).

So far, there are no indications that relevant differences exist between the various β-adrenoceptor blocking agents with respect to the treatment of cardiac arrhythmia. Obviously, properties like β_1-selectivity, membrane stabilization, and ISA are not of major importance for the antiarrhythmic activity of the β-adrenoceptor blockers.

More recently, β-blockers have proved to be of value in secondary prevention after myocardial infarction, with the aim to reduce the incidence of death and reinfarction. This protective effect has been demonstrated for timolol, metoprolol, propranolol, and sotalol (17–20). The only property common to these compounds is their ability to block β_1-adrenoceptors. As yet, no arguments have been introduced for the view that properties like β-selectivity and membrane stabilization are relevant for the cardioprotective effect.

For the sake of completeness, it should be mentioned that β-blockers may be of potential use in the following cardiovascular disorders: impending myocardial infarction; acute myocardial infarction, with the aim to reduce the size of the infarction; dissecting aortic aneurysm (maintenance therapy with a β-blocker after rapid lowering of blood pressure); asymmetric septum hypertrophy, through reduction of the gradient between the left ventricle and aorta, accompanied by a favourable influence on the induction of ventricular arrhythmia; and Fallot's tetralogy, owing to a reduction of spasm in the outflow tract of the right ventricle during a cyanotic spell. The detailed positions of the β-blockers in these conditions remain to be established. Moreover, no information exists with respect to a possible preference of particular properties of the β-blockers (selectivity, ISA) in these cardiological disorders.

Neurology and psychiatry

β-Adrenoceptor blocking drugs may be of use in the following situations (15): chronic migraine; anxiety combined with tachycardia; and certain forms of tremor. The treatment of migraine with β-blockers is empirical. So far, there is only a reasonable degree of experience with propranolol. A β_2-effect appears to be involved. In the treatment of anxiety with a β-blocker, it seems likely, although not proven, that the inhibition of tachycardia by a peripheral effect disrupts a vicious cycle, thus diminishing the facilitative influence of palpitations on anxiety. However, a direct central effect of the β-blockers is difficult to rule out entirely. The antianxiety effect of the β-blockers is the basis of their application as a kind of doping in certain sports (target shooting, motor car racing). A systematic study of different β-blockers in these conditions has not yet been carried out (15).

The antitremor effect of β-blockers is due to the blockade of β_2-adrenoceptors located on skeletal muscle. The β_1-effect is probably not relevant to the antitremor effect. For this purpose, more or less selective β_2-adrenoceptor blocking agents are being developed at present by the pharmaceutical industry. ICI 118,551 (21) is an example of such a compound.

Ophthalmology

Treatment of glaucoma simplex can be carried out with local application of timolol or other β-blocking drugs, provided that they are not local anaesthetic agents (15). The topical application of local anaesthetic agents to the eye, particularly for a prolonged period, inhibits the corneal reflex and hence may lead to irritation and infection. The lowering of ocular pressure by a β-adrenoceptor blocker is probably a β_2-effect (22). The blockade of β_2-adrenoceptors inhibits the production of ocular fluid, without greatly affecting its outflow. Timolol is the most important β-blocker so far marketed as eye drops for the treatment of glaucoma, but recently metipranolol has been introduced for the same purpose.

Endocrine disorders

β-Blockers can be of use in the non-surgical treatment of hyperthyroidism, particularly with respect to the treatment of cardiac arrhythmia in this condition, which is based on enhanced cardiac sensitivity for catecholamines. Also, in a thyrotoxic crisis (storm), β-adrenoceptor blocking drugs display beneficial effects. The interference of these drugs with the conversion of thyroxine into tri-iodothyronine has been discussed as a potential beneficial effect of β-adrenoceptor blocking agents in this condition (15). As a rule, the non-selective blocker propranolol is used for this purpose. The roles of β_1 selectivity, membrane stabilization, and ISA in this connection have not been studied systematically.

Side effects and contraindications; interactions with other drugs

Side-effects

Most of the side-effects of β-adrenoceptor blockers are due to the blockade of β_1- and/or β_2-adrenoceptors. Well-known side effects caused by the blockade of β-adrenoceptors include (7,8): obstructive airways disease (β_2); untreated congestive heart failure (β_1); impaired AV conduction with bradycardia (β_1): reduced rate of sinus node firing with bradycardia (β_1); and hypoglycaemia ($\beta_2 > \beta_1$). The well-known complaint of cold extremities is due to vasoconstriction secondary to the blockade of vascular β_2-adrenoceptors, thus allowing unimpaired vasoconstriction induced by the stimulation of vascular α-adrenoceptors. The aforementioned indications concerning the receptor type involved would suggest that all typical cardiac side-effects (congestive heart failure, bradycardia, impaired AV conduction) are bound to occur for all β-blockers, irrespective of any β_1-selective potency or not. ISA might be of theoretical advantage with respect to the development of congestive heart failure and bradycardia, but in practice this advantage is marginal and probably not clinically relevant. It should be expected that β_1 selectivity would cause less obvious hypoglycaemia and less intense peripheral vasoconstriction. Indeed, it has been observed in clinical practice that these two types of side-effects are less severe for β_1-selective drugs than for the non-selective $\beta_1 + \beta_2$-receptor blocking agents. The influence of β-adrenoreceptor blocking agents with various properties on plasma glucose and lipids was discussed in some detail by Van Brummelen (23).

Similarly, it should be anticipated that β_1-selective drugs cause less severe bronchoconstriction than the non-selective drugs. This may be true in animal models and in hypertensive patients with a healthy airways system. However, in patients suffering from obstructive airways disease, the β_1-selective drugs can also cause bronchoconstriction and impaired ventilation, possibly because the selectivity of the so-called cardioselective drugs developed until now is limited, with some β_2-effect still being present. Moreover, bronchoconstriction may, to some degree, also be mediated by β_1-adrenoceptors and not exclusively by β_2-receptors (24). On the other hand, it was discussed recently by Van Herwaarden (24) that β-blockers with ISA cause somewhat less intense impairment of ventilation than do drugs devoid of this property.

The aforementioned side-effects, based on β_1- and/or β_2-receptor blockade, may also be observed with topical application of β-blockers to the eye in the treatment of glaucoma. In particular, bradycardia and bronchoconstriction should be anticipated. Hallucinations and vivid dreams have been observed as central nervous side-effects. An unspecific feeling of fatigue and reduced capability to exercise are more common side-effects that are at least partly based on central nervous mechanisms. These side-effects often become particularly noticeable to the patient when the treatment with the β-blocker is interrupted.

It remains unclear whether these central nervous system side-effects are related to either β_1- or β_2-receptor blockade or both. One would expect an obvious relationship with the ability of the drugs to penetrate the brain. However, in practice, the hydrophilic β-blockers, which less readily penetrate, also cause these central nervous system side-effects. Apart from the more or less specific side-effects discussed above, β-blockers can also cause less well-defined adverse reactions, like gastrointestinal discomfort and allergic reactions, which are probably not specifically related to β-receptor blockade. Allergic reactions are particularly observed around the eye when the drug is applied topically in the treatment of glaucoma. The deleterious oculomucocutaneous syndrome observed for practolol has not so far been reported for other β-blockers. This syndrome is unrelated to β-adrenoceptor blockade.

Contraindications

Obstructive airways disease is an obvious contraindication for β-adrenoceptor blockers. The β_1-selective drugs and those possessing ISA are probably less dangerous but certainly not safe in these conditions. For details see Van Herwaarden (24).

Uncompensated congestive heart failure, bradycardia, and impaired AV conduction are also contraindications for β-adrenoceptor blockers. The problems are caused by β_1-adrenoceptor blockade. Accordingly, these contraindications hold for all β-blockers so far developed, properties like selectivity, ISA, and membrane stabilization being irrelevant. β-Blockers should be used reluctantly in patients with peripheral vascular disease leading to ischaemia, both in atherosclerotic disorders and in particular in conditions with a vasospastic component, such as Raynaud's phenomenon. The β_1-selective compounds are preferable in such a situation, since they cause less peripheral vasoconstriction than the non-selective drugs that also block β_2-adrenoceptors (7).

Interactions with other drugs

β-Blockers can be combined with various types of other drugs, usually without causing relevant interactions. However, problems may arise when β-adrenoceptor blocking agents are applied simultaneously with insulin and oral antidiabetics and calcium entry blockers.

β-Adrenoceptor blocking agents will enhance the hypoglycaemic effect induced by insulin and oral antidiabetics. The hypoglycaemia caused by β-blockers is mediated by a β_2-effect. For this reason it seems preferable that a diabetic patient, who is being treated with insulin or an oral antidiabetic agent and who requires a β-adrenoceptor blocker, receives a β_1-selective agent like atenolol or metoprolol instead of a non-selective agent that simultaneously blocks β_1-adrenoceptors. Other characteristics such as membrane stabilization and ISA are probably not relevant in this respect.

Calcium entry blockers of the verapamil type and β-adrenoceptor blocking agents both depress cardiac frequency, AV conduction, and contractility, although via different mechanisms. From a theoretical point of view, it would therefore seem unwise to combine both groups of drugs. However, an absolute contraindication for the combination of a β-blocker and a calcium entry blocker does not necessarily exist. Nifedipine and β-adrenoceptor blocking agents are frequently combined in the treatment of angina, and in the majority of patients this combination is effective and not problematic, although enhanced congestive heart failure caused by such a combination has been reported in a few cases (25).

Caution should be maintained, however, when verapamil and a β-blocker are applied simultaneously. In contrast to nifedipine, verapamil also has a depressant effect on cardiac contractility, heart rate and AV conduction. As such, there is an additive action in combination with a β-adrenoceptor blocking agent. The interaction between both drugs is probably most relevant when a patient who is regularly treated with an orally administered β-blocker is to receive an intravenous dose of verapamil. Combined oral treatment with both drugs in moderate doses does not, however, pose particular problems and even appears to be greatly beneficial in exercise-induced angina.

Finally, with respect to the combination of β-adrenoceptor blocking agents and other drugs, it should be mentioned that the withdrawal symptoms observed after abrupt cessation of treatment with clonidine are significantly enhanced by a β-adrenoceptor blocking agent. This interaction, which is rare, reflects the unopposed α-receptor stimulation brought about by the clonidine withdrawal phenomenon.

Characteristics of bopindolol

The characteristics of the new β-adrenoceptor blocking agent bopindolol (LT 31–200; [4(2-benzoyloxy-3-tert. butylaminopropoxy)-2-methylindole hydrogen-malonate]) are the subject of most of the papers in this publication. For further details these characteristics may be briefly summarized as follows (26–30): bopindolol is a potent β-adrenoceptor blocking agent, which blocks both β_1- and β_2-adrenoceptors. As such it is a non-specific blocker. In animal experiments it displays a certain degree of ISA, in other words bopindolol may be called a potential agonist. A further characteristic of bopindolol is its slow onset and unusually long duration of action. The slow onset of its effect is caused by the fact that bopindolol is a pro-drug. *In vivo* it is hydrolyzed to yield benzoic acid and the active β-adrenoceptor blocker.

References

(1) Timmermans PBMWM, van Zwieten PA. The postsynaptic α_2-adrenoceptor. *J Auton Pharmacol* 1981; **1**: 171–183.
(2) Frishman W. Clinical pharmacology of the new beta-adrenergic blocking drugs. Part 1. Pharmacodynamic and pharmacokinetic properties. *Am Heart J* 1979; **97**: 663–670.
(3) Nahorski SR. Identification and significance of beta-adrenoceptor subtypes. *TIPS* 1981; **3**: 95–98.
(4) Ruffolo RR, Spradin TA, Pollack GD. *et al.* Alpha and beta adrenergic effect of the stereoisomers of dobutamine. *J Pharmacol Exp Ther* 1981; **219**: 447–452.
(5) Frishman WH, β-Adrenoceptor antagonists: New drugs and new indications. *N Engl J Med* 1981; **305**: 500–506.
(6) McDevitt DG, β-adrenoceptor antagonists and respiratory function. *Br J Clin Pharmacol* 1981; **5**: 97–99.
(7) Opie LH, Drugs and the heart. I. Beta-blocking agents. *Lancet* 1980; **i**: 693–699.
(8) Frishman W, Silverman R. Clinical pharmacology of the new beta-adrenergic blocking drugs. Part 2. Physiological and metabolic effects. *Am Heart J* 1979; **97**: 797–806.
(9) Ariëns EJ. Intrinsic activity: partial agonists and partial antagonists. *J Cardiovasc Pharmacol* 1983; **5** (Suppl 1): S8–S15.
(10) Weinstock M. The presynaptic effect of β-adrenoceptor antagonists on noradrenergic neurones. *Life Sci* 1976; **19**: 1453–1466.
(11) Svendsen TL. Central hemodynamics of β-adrenoceptor blocking drugs: β_1-selectivity versus intrinsic sympathomimetic activity. *J Cardiovasc Pharmacol* 1983; **5** (Suppl 1): S21–S25.
(12) Hansson L, Svensson A, Gudbrandsson T, Sivertsson R. Treatment of hypertension with β-blockers with and without intrinsic sympathomimetic activity. *J Cardiovasc Pharmacol* 1983; **5** (Suppl 1): S26–S29.
(13) Thadani U, Davidson C, Singleton W. *et al.* Comparison of the immediate effects of five β-adrenoceptor blocking drugs with different ancillary properties in angina pectoris. *N Eng J Med* 1979; **300**: 750–755.
(14) Van Ekelen WAAJ, Robles de Medina EO. Coronary arterial spasm and its treatment. *Progr Pharmacol* 1981; **4**: 43–49.
(15) Frishman W, Silverman R. Clinical pharmacology of the new beta-adrenergic blocking drugs. Part 3. Comparative clinical experience and new therapeutic applications. *Am Heart J* 1979; **98**: 119–130.
(16) Wit AL, Hoffman BF, Rosen MR. Electrophysiology and pharmacology of cardiac arrhythmias. IX. Cardiac electrophysiologic effects of beta adrenergic receptor stimulation and blockade. Part B. *Am Heart J* 1975; **90**: 665–674.

(17) The Norwegian Multicenter Study Group. Timolol-induced reduction in mortality and reinfarction in patients surviving acute myocardial infarction. *N Engl J Med* 1981; **304**: 801–807.

(18) Hjalmarson Å, Herlitz J, Málek I. *et al.* Effect on mortality of metoprolol in acute myocardial infarction. *Lancet* 1981; **ii**: 823–827.

(19) β-Blocker Heart Attack Study Group. The β-blocker heart attack trial. *JAMA* 1981; **246**: 2073–2074.

(20) Julian DG, Prescott RJ, Jackson FS. *et al.* Controlled trial of sotalol for one year after myocardial infarction. *Lancet* 1982; **i**: 1142–1148.

(21) Bilski A, Dorries S, Fitzgerald JD. *et al.* ICI 118,551, a potent β-adrenoceptor antagonist. *Br J Pharmacol* 1980; **69**: 292P–293P.

(22) Innemee HC, van Zwieten PA. The role of β_2-adrenoceptors in the IOP-lowering effect of adrenaline. *Av Graefes Arch Clin Exp Ophthalmol* 1982; **218**: 297–300.

(23) Van Brummelen P. The relevance of intrinsic sympathomimetic activity for β-blocker-induced changes in plasma lipids. *J Cardiovasc Pharmacol* 1983; **5**(Suppl 1): S51–S55.

(24) Van Herwaarden CLA. β-Adrenoceptor blockade and pulmonary function in patients suffering from chronic obstructive lung disease. *J Cardiovasc Pharmacol* 1983; **5**(Suppl 1): S46–S50.

(25) Robson RH, Vishwanath MC. Nifedipine and beta blockade as a cause of cardiac failure. *Br Med J* 1982; **284**: 104.

(26) Berthold R, Waite R, Weber H. Pharmacological studies with bopindolol: a new long acting β-adrenoceptor antagonist. *Br J Pharmacol* 1981; **74**: 829P.

(27) Aellig WH. Duration of action and plasma levels of beta-adrenoceptor blocking drugs. *Arch Int Pharmacodyn Ther* 1980; (suppl): 32–37.

(28) Aellig WH. Clinical pharmacological experiments with bopindolol (LT 31-200): a long acting β-adrenoceptor blocking drug with partial agonist activity. *Br J Clin Pharmacol* 1982; **13**: 267P–268P.

(29) Aellig WH. Pharmacological experiments in healthy volunteers with bopindolol, a long-acting β-adrenoceptor blocking drug with partial agonist activity. *Br J Clin Pharmacol* 1985; **19**: 775–781.

(30) Aellig WH, Nüesch E, Engel G, Grevel J, Niederberger W, Rosenthaler J. Relationship between plasma concentrations and cardiac β-adrenoceptor blockade—a study with oral and intravenous bopindolol. *Br J Clin Pharmacol* 1986; **21**: 45–51.

Reduction in lymphocyte β_2-adrenoceptor density, caused by β-adrenoceptor antagonists with ISA: a possible explanation for the absence of 'rebound-effects'

O. GALAL, X. L. WANG and O.-E. BRODDE

Biochemical Research Laboratories, Medical Clinic and Policlinic, Division of Renal and Hypertensive Diseases, University Hospital Essen, Essen, Federal Republic of Germany

Summary

In order to study the role of intrinsic sympathomimetic activity (ISA) in β-adrenoceptor antagonist-induced modulation of β-adrenoceptor function, in healthy volunteers the effects of propranolol (non-selective β-adrenoceptor antagonist *without* ISA) and pindolol (non-selective β-adrenoceptor antagonist *with* ISA) on lymphocyte β_2-adrenoceptor density (assessed by $(-)-{}^{125}$I-iodocyanopindolol binding) were compared with those of the non-selective β-adrenoceptor antagonist bopindolol *with* ISA, the β_1-selective antagonists bisoprolol *without* ISA and celiprolol *with* ISA and the β_2-selective antagonist ICI 118 551 *without* ISA. The ISA of the β-adrenoceptor antagonists was determined on the spontaneously beating right atrium of reserpinized rats (ISA isoprenaline = 1·0). Propranolol (*no* ISA, 4 × 40 mg/day for 8 days) increased lymphocyte β_2-adrenoceptor density by about 35–40%; after withdrawal β_2-adrenoceptor density returned slowly to control being still significantly elevated after 3 days. A similar increase in lymphocyte β_2-adrenoceptor density was observed during treatment with the β_2-selective antagonist ICI 118 551 (*no* ISA, 3 × 25 mg/day), while the β_1-selective antagonist bisoprolol (*no* ISA, 1 × 10 mg/day) did not affect lymphocyte β_2-adrenoceptor density. On the contrary, administration of β-adrenoceptor antagonists *with* ISA (pindolol, non-selective, ISA = 0·39; 2 × 5 mg/day; bopindolol, non-selective, ISA = 0·27, 1 × 2 mg/day; celiprolol, β_1-selective, ISA = 0·32, 1 × 200 mg/day) caused decreases in lymphocyte β_2-adrenoceptor density, whereby the magnitude in β_2-adrenoceptor reduction is obviously depending on the strength of the ISA: pindolol (– 50%) produced greater β_2-adrenoceptor decreases than celiprolol (– 30%) or bopindolol (– 35%) as is the

The position of bopindolol, a new β-blocker, edited by P. A. van Zwieten, 1987: Royal Society of Medicine Services International Congress and Symposium Series No. 106, published by Royal Society of Medicine Services Limited.

ISA of pindolol greater than that of bopindolol or celiprolol. These results indicate that the ISA of β-adrenoceptor antagonists plays an important role in modulating β-adrenoceptor density and hence tissue responsiveness to β-adrenoceptor stimulation. All β-adrenoceptor antagonists *without* ISA increase β-adrenoceptor density and -responsiveness, which may lead to 'rebound effects' after abrupt withdrawal. The lack of any effect of the β_1-adrenoceptor selective antagonist bisoprolol does not contradict this assumption; it may well be that long-term treatment with bisoprolol increases subtype-selectively β_1-adrenoceptor density (for example in the heart). On the other hand, the reduction in β-adrenoceptor density and -responsiveness caused by (all) β-adrenoceptor antagonists *with* ISA—irrespective of whether they are non-selective or β_1-selective—should prevent the occurrence of 'rebound-effects' after abrupt discontinuation of treatment with these drugs.

Introduction

β-Adrenoceptor antagonists are commonly used in the therapy of hypertension (for recent reviews see Refs 1,2). There are several reports in the literature showing that abrupt discontinuation of antihypertensive therapy with propranolol (a non-selective β-adrenoceptor antagonist *without* intrinsic sympathomimetic activity (ISA)) might lead to clinical symptoms that suggest adrenergic hypersensitivity ('propranolol withdrawal phenomenon', for recent review see Ref. 3). On the other hand, rebound effects have not been observed after abrupt withdrawal of pindolol, a non-selective β-adrenoceptor antagonist *with* ISA (4,5). Obviously, the ISA plays an important role in β-adrenoceptor antagonist-induced modulation of β-adrenoceptor function.

Circulating lymphocytes containing a homogeneous population of β_2-adrenoceptors (6) excitatorily coupled to the adenylate cyclase system (7) are a frequently used model to study drug-induced alterations of β-adrenoceptors in man (for recent reviews see Refs 8,9). On this model we have compared the effects of propranolol and pindolol on β_2-adrenoceptor density (assessed by $(-)-{}^{125}$I-iodocyanopindolol (ICYP) binding) with those of the non-selective β-adrenoceptor antagonist bopindolol (10) *with* ISA, the selective β_1-adrenoceptor antagonists bisoprolol (11) *without* ISA and celiprolol (12) *with* ISA and the selective β_2-adrenoceptor antagonist ICI 118 551 (13) *without* ISA in order to further investigate the role of ISA in modulating β-adrenoceptor function in man.

Subjects and methods

53 healthy normotensive volunteers (44 males, 9 females, mean age $25{\cdot}7 \pm 1{\cdot}6$ (range 19–46) years; blood pressure averaged to $122{\cdot}8 \pm 3{\cdot}9/76{\cdot}2 \pm 3$ mmHg) participated in the study after having given informed written consent. All were drug-free and had undergone physical examination to exclude asthma, chronic pulmonary disease, diabetes mellitus, cardiac disease, and symptoms referable to the cardiovascular system. Blood samples (30 ml heparin blood for determination of β_2-adrenoceptor density in lymphocytes) were withdrawn by venipuncture between 8.00 and 10.00 h after 30 min of rest with the subjects in sitting position. The β-adrenoceptor antagonists were self-administered orally for 8 days: propranolol 4 × 40 mg/day at 6.00, 12.00, 18.00 and 24.00 h; pindolol 2 × 5 mg/day at 7.00 and 19.00 h; bisoprolol 1 × 10 mg/day, celiprolol 1 × 200 mg/day and bopindolol 1 × 2 mg/day at 19.00 h;

ICI 118 551 3×25 mg/day at 7.00, 14.00 and 21.00 h. On days 2, 4 and 8 after initiation of the β-adrenoceptor antagonist administration and on 3–4 days after withdrawal of the β-adrenoceptor antagonists blood samples were collected. Lymphocytes were isolated from heparinized blood and the β_2-adrenoceptor density was determined by ICYP binding as recently described (14,15). The ISA of the β-adrenoceptor antagonists was determined as positive chronotropic effect on spontaneously beating right atria from reserpinized rats in relationship to isoprenaline (ISA = 1·0). Details of the procedure have been described elsewhere (16,17).

Statistical evaluations

The experimental data given in the figures are means ± SEM of *n* experiments. The maximal number of ICYP binding sites and the equilibrium dissociation constant (K_D) for ICYP were calculated from plots according to Scatchard (18). The significance of differences was estimated by Student's *t*-test. A *p*-value smaller than 0·05 was considered to be significant.

Results and discussion

Intrinsic sympathomimetic activity (ISA) of the β-adrenoceptor antagonists

The ISA of the β-adrenoceptor antagonists was determined on spontaneously beating right atria of reserpinized rats (15–17). On this preparation the maximum increase in heart rate evoked by pindolol amounted to 39% of that of isoprenaline (ISA of pindolol = 0·39). Bopindolol was slightly less active (ISA = 0·27), whereas propranolol was devoid of any ISA (15–17). From the β_1- and β_2-selective antagonists studied, celiprolol exerted a strong positive chronotropic effect (ISA = 0·32), whereas bisoprolol and ICI 118 551 showed no chronotropic activity.

Effects of the β-adrenoceptor antagonists on lymphocyte β_2-adrenoceptor density

The non-selective β-adrenoceptor antagonist propranolol *without* ISA led to rapid increase in lymphocyte β_2-adrenoceptor density; 2 days after initiation of propranolol administration β_2-adrenoceptor density was already increased by about 25% (Fig. 1). β_2-Adrenoceptor density remained increased throughout the treatment period; the maximum increase was reached 8 days after initiation of treatment and amounted to approximately 40% (Fig. 1). After withdrawal of propranolol β_2-adrenoceptor density declined slowly, being still significantly increased after 3 days. The properties of lymphocyte β_2-adrenoceptors—characterized *in vitro* by radioligand binding studies (6,19,20)—are very similar to those in other peripheral and/or central tissues, including human heart (21). In addition, we have recently shown, that in man β-adrenoceptor density in circulating lymphocytes is highly significantly correlated with the corresponding β-adrenoceptor density *and* -responsiveness

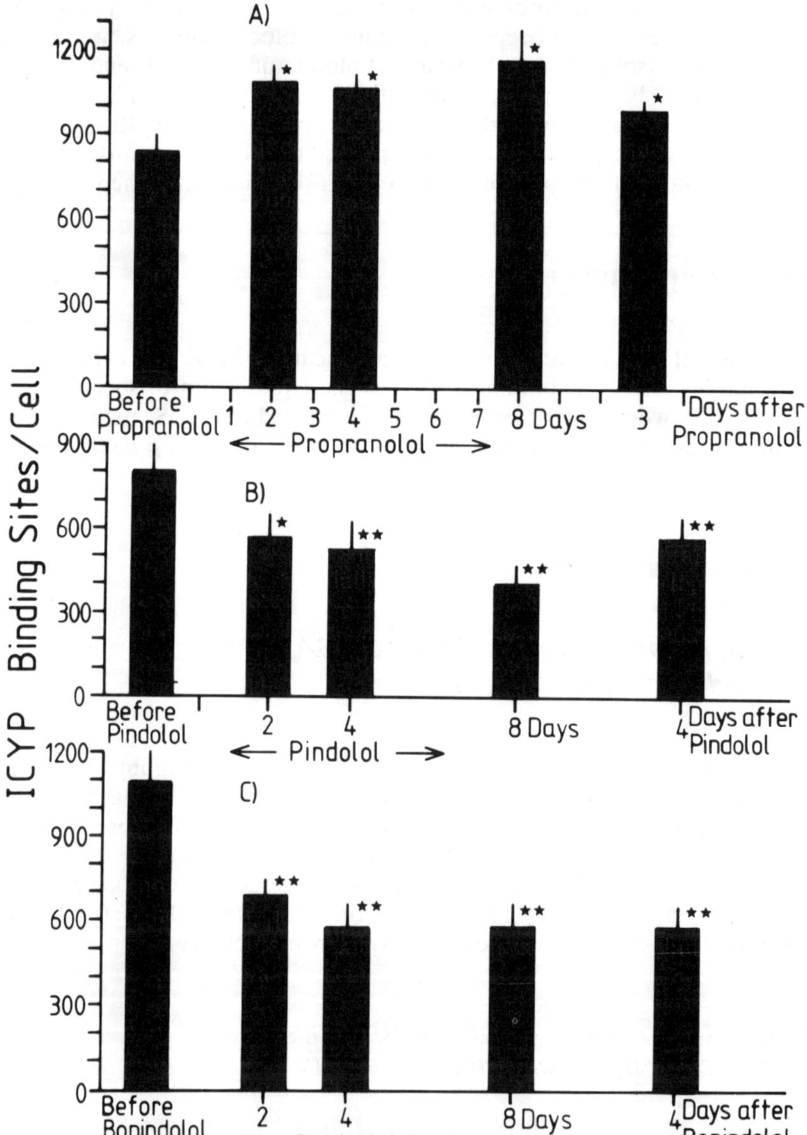

*Figure 1. Effects of non-selective β-adrenoceptor antagonist (propranolol without ISA, pindolol and bopindolol with ISA) administration on β_2-adrenoceptor density in lymphocytes of healthy volunteers. A) Propranolol (4 × 40 mg/day). B) Pindolol (2 × 5 mg/day). C) Bopindolol (1 × 2 mg/day). Ordinate: Lymphocyte β_2-adrenoceptor density — determined by Scatchard-analysis (18) of ICYP binding — in ICYP binding sites/cell. Six male volunteers (mean age: 27·0 ± 0·8 (24–30) years) participated in the propranolol study, 8 (four males, four females, mean age: 24·5 ± 1·1 (20–28) years) in the pindolol study and five (two males, three females, mean age: 25·8 ± 1·1 (22–28) years) in the bopindolol study. Given are means ± SEM **p < 0·01, *p < 0·05 vs predrug levels.*

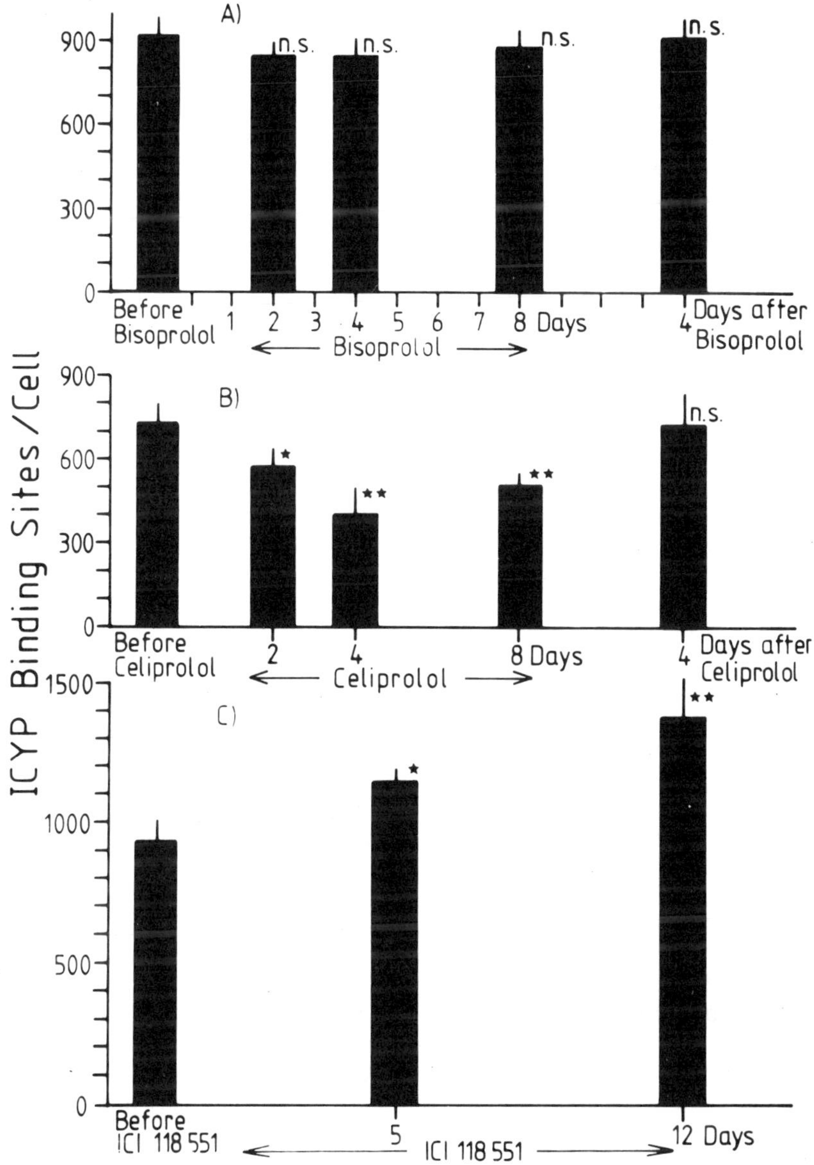

*Figure 2. Effects of β_1- (bisoprolol without ISA, celiprolol with ISA) and β_2- (ICI 118 551 without ISA) selective adrenoceptor antagonist administration on β_2-adrenoceptor density in lymphocytes of healthy volunteers. A) Bisoprolol (1 × 10 mg/day). B) Celiprolol (1 × 200 mg/day). C) ICI 118 551 (3 × 25 mg/day). Ordinate: Lymphocyte β_2-adrenoceptor density — determined by Scatchard-analysis (18) of ICYP binding — in ICYP binding sites/cell. Twelve male volunteers (mean age: 23·8 ± 1·3 (19–36) years) participated in the bisoprolol study, eight (six males, two females, mean age: 29·3 ± 3·0 (20–46) years) in the celiprolol study, and six males (mean age: 24·5 ± 1·7 (20–31) years) in the ICI 118 551 study. Given are means ± SEM **p<0·01, *p<0·05 vs predrug levels.*

(assessed as increases in contractile force induced by isoprenaline) in the right atria obtained from the same subjects (22). Thus, it might be concluded that the propranolol-induced increases in human lymphocyte β_2-adrenoceptors could mirror enhanced β-adrenoceptor responsiveness in peripheral and/or central tissues. Such an increased responsiveness of β-adrenoceptors might be the cause for the untoward side-effects observed after abrupt withdrawal of propranolol administration (3).

A similar increase in lymphocyte β_2-adrenoceptor density was observed after administration of the highly selective β_2-adrenoceptor antagonist ICI 118 551 (3×25 mg/day) *without* ISA which amounted after 5 days to 25% and after 12 days to 50% (Fig. 2). These results favour the idea that long-term treatment with all β-adrenoceptor antagonists *without* ISA should lead to increases in β-adrenoceptor density. Hence, after abrupt withdrawal of therapy with all β-adrenoceptor antagonists *without* ISA rebound effects can occur. On the other hand, the highly selective β_1-adrenoceptor antagonist bisoprolol (1×10 mg/day) *without* ISA did not affect lymphocyte β_2-adrenoceptor density (Fig. 2), neither during treatment nor after withdrawal. This indicates that changes in lymphocyte β-adrenoceptors reflect subtype selectively changes in β_2-adrenoceptors. The lack of any effect of bisoprolol on lymphocyte β_2-adrenoceptor density does not exclude the possibility that long-term treatment might increase β_1-adrenoceptors (for example in the heart) thus leading to symptoms of adrenergic hypersensitivity after withdrawal.

In contrast to the β-adrenoceptor antagonists *without* ISA the non-selective β-adrenoceptor antagonist pindolol (2×5 mg/day) *with* ISA caused decreases in β_2-adrenoceptor density in lymphocytes which were already significant 2 days after administration of the drug (Fig. 1). The maximum decrease induced by pindolol was approximately 50% (8 days after initiation of drug administration). Bopindolol (1×2 mg/day) *with* ISA (0·27) exerted similar effects as pindolol (Fig. 1): 2 days after initiation of bopindolol treatment β_2-adrenoceptor density in lymphocytes was reduced by approximately 30% and remained on this reduced level throughout the treatment period (Fig. 1). After abrupt withdrawal of pindolol as well as of bopindolol β_2-adrenoceptor density increased very slowly and was still significantly reduced 4 days after withdrawal.

Not only the non-selective β-adrenoceptor antagonists *with* ISA, but also the β_1-adrenoceptor selective antagonist celiprolol *with* ISA produced significant decreases in lymphocyte β_2-adrenoceptor density (Fig. 2). The maximum decrease in lymphocyte β_2-adrenoceptor density evoked by celiprolol was similar to that induced by bopindolol as was the ISA of celiprolol in the same range as that of bopindolol (see above). The fact that all β-adrenoceptor antagonists *with* ISA reduce β-adrenoceptor density might be of clinical importance: since no adrenergic hypersensitivity can develop, rapid cessation of drug treatment should not induce rebound effects. In fact, pindolol has been found to be devoid of any symptoms of adrenergic hypersensitivity after abrupt withdrawal (4,5).

Conclusion

The present results clearly demonstrate that the ISA plays an important role in β-adrenoceptor antagonist-induced modulation of β-adrenoceptor density. β-Adrenoceptor antagonists *without* ISA lead to increases in β-adrenoceptor density still persisting after abrupt withdrawal which might explain the 'β-blocker rebound phenomena'. Subtype selective β-adrenoceptor antagonists like bisoprolol (β_1) or ICI 118 551 (β_2), however, seem to increase subtype selectively only β_1- or

β_2-adrenoceptors, respectively, which might be favourable under certain clinical conditions. Since β-adrenoceptor antagonists *with* ISA decrease β-adrenoceptor density rebound effects should not occur after discontinuation of treatment.

References

(1) Scriabine A. β-Adrenoceptor blocking drugs in hypertension. *Ann Rev Pharmacol Toxicol* 1979; **19**: 269–284.

(2) Van Baak MA, Struyker Boudier AJ, Smits JFM. Antihypertensive mechanisms of beta-adrenoceptor blockade: a review. *Clin Exp Hypertens* 1985; **A7**: 1–72.

(3) Prichard BNC, Tomlinson B, Walden RJ, Bhattacharjee P.The β-adrenergic blockade withdrawal phenomenon. *J Cardiovasc Pharmacol* 1983; **5** (Suppl 1): S56–S62.

(4) Szecsi E, Kohlschütter S, Schiess W, Lang E. Abrupt withdrawal of pindolol or metoprolol after chronic therapy. *Br J Clin Pharmacol* 1982; **13** (Suppl 2): 353S–357S.

(5) Walden RJ, Bhattarcharjee P, Tomlinson B, Cashin J, Graham BR, Prichard BNC. The effect of intrinsic sympathomimetic activity on β-receptor responsiveness after β-adrenoceptor blockade withdrawal. *Br J Clin Pharmacol* 1982; **13** (Suppl 2): 359S–364S.

(6) Brodde O-E, Engel G, Hoyer D, Bock KD, Weber F. The β-adrenergic receptor in human lymphocytes: Subclassification by the use of a new radio-ligand, $(\pm)-{}^{125}$I-iodocyanopindolol. *Life Sci* 1981; **29**: 2189–2198.

(7) Brodde O-E, Daul AE, O'Hara N, Khalifa AM. Properties of α- and β-adrenoceptors in circulating blood cells of patients with essential hypertension. *J Cardiovasc Pharmacol* 1985; **7** (Suppl 6): S162–S167.

(8) Motulsky HJ, Insel PA. Adrenergic receptors in man. Direct identification, physiologic regulation and clinical alterations. *N Engl J Med* 1982; **307**: 18–29.

(9) Stiles GL, Caron MG, Lefkowitz RJ. β-Adrenergic receptors: biochemical mechanisms of physiological regulation. *Physiol Rev* 1984; **64**: 661–743.

(10) Schiess W, Welzel D, Gugler R. Double-blind comparison of once-daily bopindolol, pindolol and atenolol in essential hypertension. *Eur J Clin Pharmacol* 1984; **27**: 529–534.

(11) Wang XL, Brinkmann M, Brodde O-E. Selective labelling of β_1-adrenoceptors in rabbit lung membranes by $(-)-{}^3$H$-$bisoprolol. *Eur J Pharmacol* 1985; **114**: 157–165.

(12) Van Inwegen RG, Khandwala A, Weinryb I, Pruss TB, Neiss E, Sutherland CA. Effects of celiprolol (REV 5320), a new cardioselective beta-adrenoceptor antagonist, on *in vitro* adenylate cyclase, alpha- and beta-adrenergic receptor binding and lipolysis. *Arch Int Pharmacodyn Ther* 1984; **272**: 40–55.

(13) Bilski AJ, Halliday SE, Fitzgerald JD, Wale JL. The pharmacology of a β_2-selective adrenoceptor antagonist (ICI 118,551). *J Cardiovasc Pharmacol* 1983; **5**: 430–437.

(14) Brodde O-E, Brinkmann M, Schemuth R, O'Hara N, Daul A. Terbutaline-induced desensitization of human lymphocyte β_2-adrenoceptors. Accelerated restoration of β-adrenoceptor responsiveness by prednisone and ketotifen. *J Clin Invest* 1985; **76**: 1096–1101.

(15) Brodde O-E, Schemuth R, Brinkmann M, Wang XL, Daul A, Borchard U. β-Adrenoceptor antagonists (non-selective as well as β_1-selective) with partial agonistic activity decrease β_2-adrenoceptor density in human lymphocytes. Evidence for a β_2-agonistic component of the partial agonistic activity. *Naunyn-Schmiedeberg's Arch Pharmacol* 1986; **333**: 130–138.

(16) Brodde O-E, Daul A, Stuka N, O'Hara N, Borchard U. Effects of β-adrenoceptor antagonist administration on β_2-adrenoceptor density in human lymphocytes. The role of the 'intrinsic sympathomimetic activity'. *Naunyn-Schmiedeberg's Arch Pharmacol* 1985; **328**: 417–422.

(17) Borchard U, Hafner D, Hirth C. In vitro studies on the pharmacological properties of diacetolol, the major metabolite of acebutolol in man. *Arch Int Pharmacodyn Ther* 1985; **273**: 4–17.
(18) Scatchard G. The attraction of proteins for small molecules and ions. *Ann N Y Acad Sci* 1949; **51**: 660–672.
(19) Williams LT, Snyderman R, Lefkowitz RJ. Identification of beta-adrenergic receptors in human lymphocytes by $(-)-{}^{3}$H-alprenolol binding. *J Clin Invest* 1976; **57**: 149–155.
(20) Galant SP, Underwood S, Duriseti L, Insel PA. Characterization of high affinity β_2-adrenergic receptor binding of $(-)-{}^{3}$H-dihydroalprenolol to human polymorphonuclear cell particulates. *J Lab Clin Med* 1978; **92**: 613–618.
(21) Brodde O-E, Karad K, Zerkowski H-R, Rohm N, Reidemeister J Chr. Coexistence of β_1- and β_2-adrenoceptors in human right atrium. Direct identification by $(\pm)-{}^{125}$ iodocyanopindolol binding. *Circ Res* 1983; **53**: 752–758.
(22) Brodde O-E, Kretsch R, Ikezono K, Zerkowski H-R, Reidemeister J Chr. Human β-adrenoceptors: relation of myocardial and lymphocyte β-adrenoceptor density. *Science* 1986; **231**: 1584–1585.

β-Blockers in hypertension

A. J. MAN IN 'T VELD

Department of Internal Medicine I, University Hospital Dijkzigt, Erasmus University, Rotterdam, The Netherlands

Summary

Over 20 years ago it was established for the first time that β-blockers could reduce high blood pressure. Since then it has been found that the balance of efficacy, safety and tolerability has caused these agents to be regarded as the drugs of choice in the treatment of hypertension. Currently, several β-blockers with different ancillary properties are available. They all have the property in common of blocking β_1-receptors, but differ from each other in a number of other respects: the incapacity of blocking β_2-receptors in low doses (β_1-receptor selectivity), the presence or absence of partial agonist activity, also known as intrinsic sympathomimetic activity (ISA), and the degree to which they are soluble in fat (lipophilicity). β_1-Selectivity is of importance in patients with obstructive lung disease requiring simultaneous treatment with a β_2-mimetic agent and in patients with type I diabetes mellitus. However, β_1-selectivity might also constitute a drawback in situations in which there is a high level of circulating adrenaline (stress, hypoglycaemia, myocardial infarction, cerebrovascular accident, anaesthesia), since in these cases the acute hypokalaemia brought about by adrenaline (β_2-effect) is suppressed much less than during non-selective β-blockade. In patients with pronounced 'central' side-effects (dreams, insomnia, hallucinations, depression, concentration disturbances), a hydrophilic β-blocker may bring relief. β-Blockers with adequate ISA exert less negative inotropic and chronotropic effect on the heart. Unlike β-blockers without ISA, these agents reduce the blood pressure by lowering the increased vascular resistance in hypertension. Additional α-adrenoceptor blockade results in a comparable haemodynamic profile. The β-blockers with ISA exert a favourable effect on the HDL/LDL-cholesterol ratio, and the so-called β-blocker withdrawal syndrome does not occur with this category. Although all β-blockers are equally effective as far as their effect on the blood pressure is concerned, it is not known whether they also exert an identical effect on the raised cardiovascular risk associated with hypertension. However, sound knowledge of the various properties of β-blockers will lead to discriminating use of these agents, resulting in an optimal balance of efficacy, safety and tolerability for the individual patient. Ultimately, this may lead to better compliance and consequently to a better prognosis.

The position of bopindolol, a new β-blocker, edited by P. A. van Zwieten, 1987: Royal Society of Medicine Services International Congress and Symposium Series No. 106, published by Royal Society of Medicine Services Limited.

Introduction

The β-blockers were originally developed for the treatment of angina pectoris and cardiac arrhythmias (1). In 1964, Prichard observed that pronethalol reduced blood pressure in a few hypertensive patients being treated with this drug because of angina pectoris (2). At present, there are several β-blockers on the market with different ancillary properties (Table 1). The relatively favourable balance of efficacy, safety and tolerability of these agents has made them into the drugs of choice in the treatment of hypertension (3).

Although all β-blockers currently available share the capacity of blocking β_1-receptors, they differ in many other respects. The most relevant additional properties of the β-blockers are:

1. a relative selectivity for β_1-receptors, also incorrectly called 'cardioselectivity',
2. presence or absence of a certain degree of partial agonist activity (PAA) also known as intrinsic sympathomimetic activity (ISA),
3. the degree of solubility in fats, which is decisive for the rate at which a β-blocker penetrates into the central nervous system and which is known as 'lipophilicity' (4–12). The most relevant consequences of these properties are discussed below.

Table 1

Ancillary properties of β-blockers

Name	ISA	β_1-Selectivity	α-Blockade	lipophilicity
Pindolol	+ + +	−	−	+
Oxprenolol	+	−	−	+ +
Alprenolol	+	−	−	+ +
Acebutolol	±	+	−	+
Penbutolol	±	−	−	+
Bopindolol	±	−	−	+
Betaxolol	−	+ +	−	+ +
Atenolol	−	+	−	−
Metoprolol	−	+	−	+ +
Propranolol	−	−	−	+ + +
Timolol	−	−	−	+ +
Sotalol	−	−	−	−
Labetalol	−	−	+	+ +

ISA = intrinsic sympathomimetic activity

Haemodynamic effects

Acute and chronic effects

In a recent study of the literature, the acute and chronic haemodynamic effects of ten β-blockers were compared (13–15). As Fig. 1 shows, in spite of major pharmacological differences, the various β-blockers have hardly any acute effect, and an identical chronic effect on blood pressure. In this respect, therefore, there is little to choose among the various representatives of this category of drugs. In addition it was found that there exists an inverse proportionality between the acute and chronic

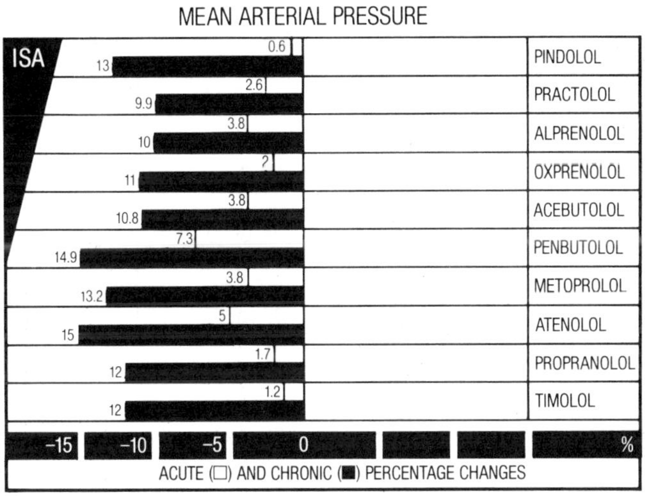

Figure 1. Acute and chronic effects of ten β-blockers in supine resting hypertensive subjects. The sequence of the drugs is depicted according to a decreasing degree of ISA. Metoprolol, atenolol, propranolol and timolol do not possess ISA.

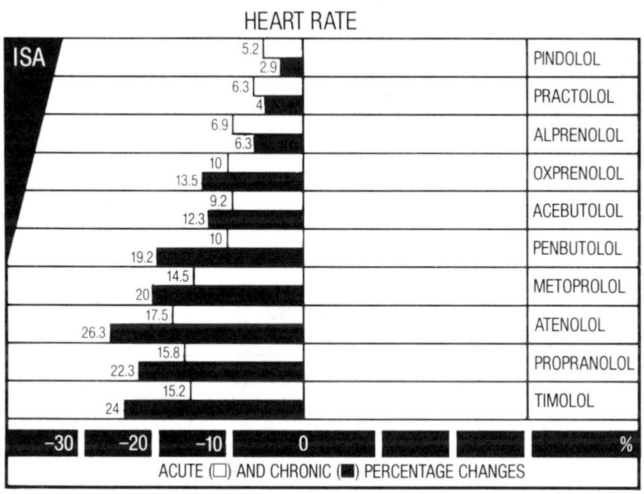

Figure 2. See legend to Fig. 1.

reduction of heart rate (Fig. 2), cardiac output (Fig. 3) and stroke volume (Fig. 5) on one hand, and the extent to which a particular β-blocker possesses ISA on the other. Since after acute administration of the various β-blockers blood pressure changes little if at all, the peripheral resistance, which in hypertension is increased in any case, will increase further in proportion to the decrease of the cardiac output (Fig. 4). It was also observed that where this reflectory increase of vascular resistance is concerned, there is no difference between selective and non-selective β-blockers. Apparently, whether the vascular β_2-receptor is or is not blocked (the so-called unopposed α-effect) plays no part in this phenomenon. The short- and long-term effects of a particular β-blocker on cardiac output are found to show hardly any difference (Fig. 3). Since meanwhile blood pressure has decreased, this decrease must be secondary to a decrease of peripheral vascular resistance. However, since initially

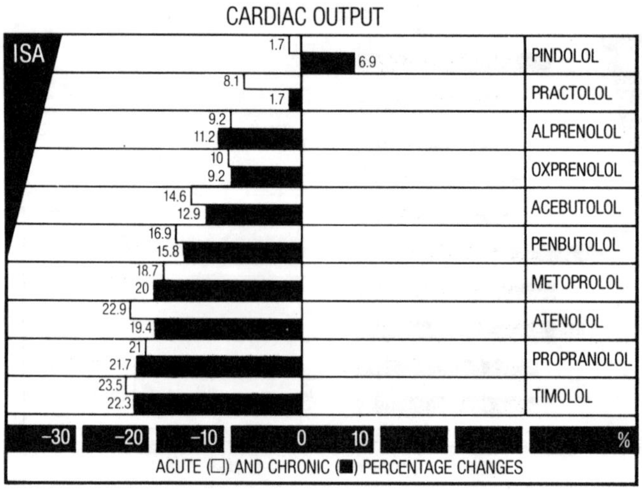

Figure 3. See legend to Fig. 1.

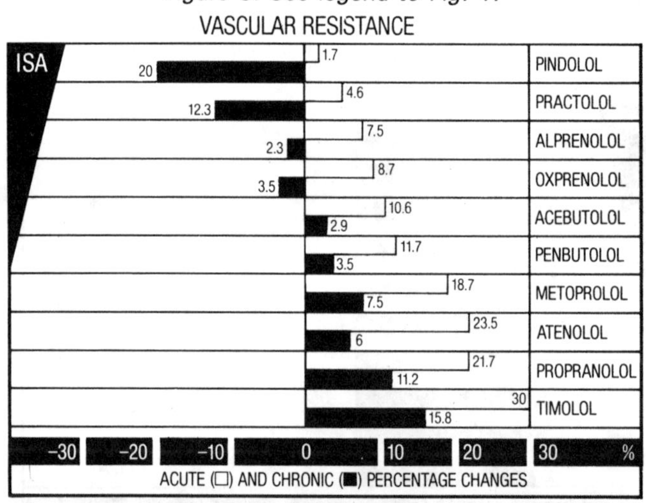

Figure 4. See legend to Fig. 1.

the vascular resistance is higher when a β-blocker has little or no ISA, a considerable difference in the absolute level of peripheral resistance will also persist in the long run. The acute effects of the various β-blockers on cardiac output are somewhat more pronounced than their effects on heart rate (Figs 2 and 3). Accordingly, stroke volume also decreases (Fig. 5). Stroke volume decreases more when little or no ISA is present. If during chronic treatment, blood pressure and vascular resistance decrease, stroke volume increases again.

Haemodynamic patterns

By definition, the cardiac output and the vascular resistance are inversely proportional to each other (Figs 6 and 7), both acutely and chronically. The increase in vascular

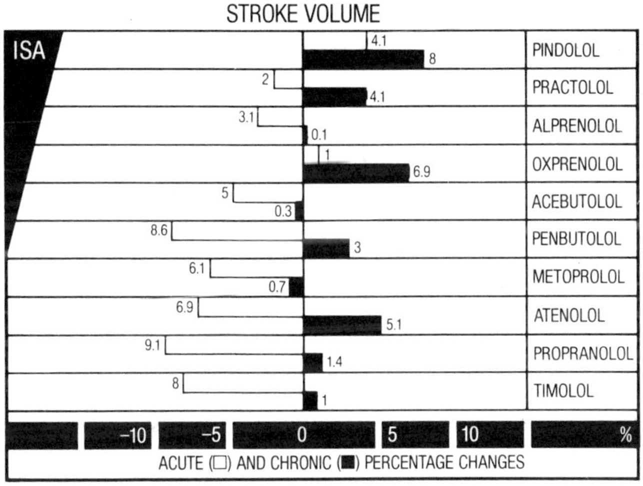

Figure 5. See legend to Fig. 1.

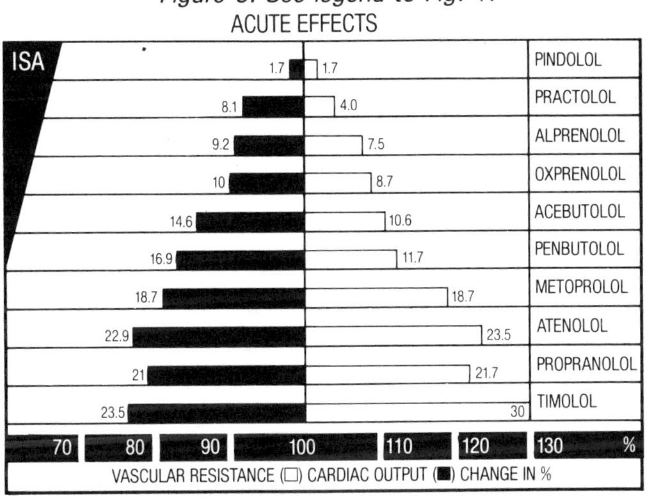

Figure 6. Interrelation between the acute changes in cardiac output and the acute changes in vascular resistance after intravenous β-blockade.

resistance due to reduction of cardiac output is not different for selective and non-selective β-blockers. With all β-blockers, the fall of the blood pressure is a consequence of a decrease of vascular resistance. Because of the lower starting value of vascular resistance during treatment with β-blockers with ISA, vascular resistance in the long run will also remain lower than on the β-blockers without this ancillary property.

The background of the fall of stroke volume after acute β-blockade is shown in Fig. 8. There exists an inversely proportional relationship between the extent of decrease of stroke volume and the extent of increase of peripheral resistance. This suggests that the combination of decreased cardiac contractility due to the β-blockade and increased vascular resistance (=afterload) are responsible for this inverse correlation. β-Blockers with a substantial amount of ISA, cause no cardiodepression and consequently, they do not trigger a reflectory increase of vascular resistance. This assumption is corroborated by the fact that the fall in vascular resistance, that is

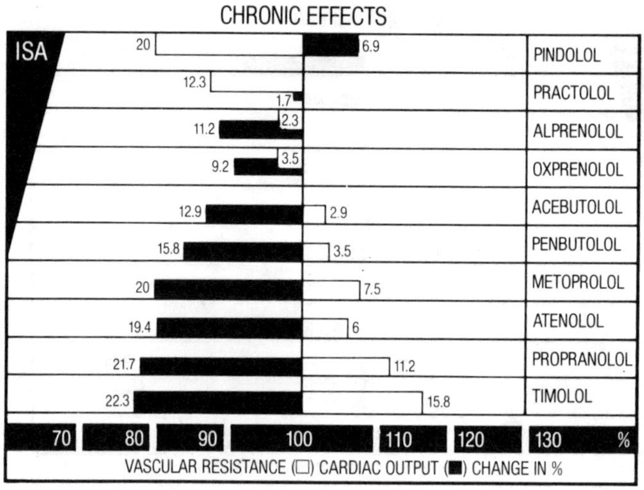

Figure 7. Interrelation between the long-term changes in cardiac output and the long-term changes in vascular resistance during oral treatment with β-blockers.

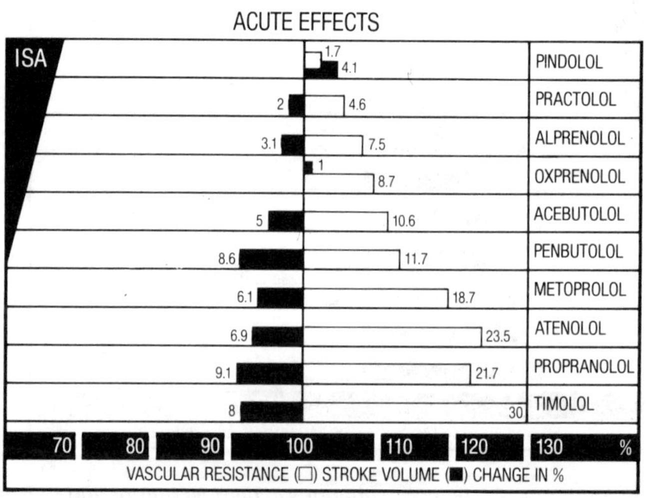

Figure 8. Interrelation between the acute changes in stroke volume and the acute changes in vascular resistance after intravenous β-blockade.

the cause of the fall of blood pressure with the various β-blockers, is associated with an increase in stroke volume (Fig. 9).

The long-term haemodynamic profile of labetalol corresponds to that of a β-blocker with strong ISA; cardiac output does not change and the raised peripheral resistance in hypertension decreases. This is due to the α_1-blocking property of labetalol which counteracts a reflectory increase of peripheral resistance, thereby causing vasodilation, while the β-blockade suppresses the reflectory tachycardia which might otherwise be expected. Accordingly, labetalol, unlike the other β-blockers, does acutely reduce blood pressure. This may be useful in acute situations, such as in patients with a phaeochromocytoma. In patients with essential hypertension, on the other hand, this should not be regarded as an advantage because too abrupt a fall in blood pressure may cause problems such as orthostatic disorders of the cerebral perfusion, with the risk of collapse.

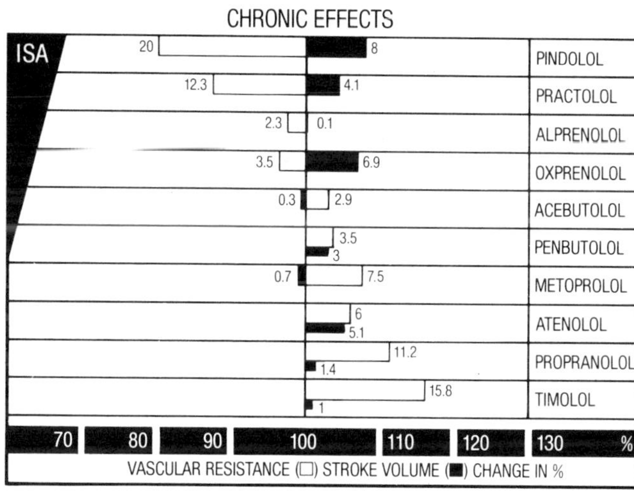

Figure 9. Interrelation between the long-term changes in stroke volume and the long-term changes in vascular resistance during oral treatment with β-blockers.

Pathophysiological consideration

From the haemodynamic point of view, hypertension of longer standing is characterized by raised peripheral resistance and a normal or decreased cardiac output. Where heart rate is concerned, there is no difference between hypertensive and normotensive subjects. Consequently, in hypertension stroke volume is normal to subnormal.

The literature shows that β-blockers without ISA hardly affect the haemodynamic abnormalities in hypertension: the peripheral resistance remains increased and even rises further, while stroke volume remains subnormal (Fig. 10). The situation is clearly different during treatment with a β-blocker with sufficient ISA to prevent a decrease of cardiac output at rest. In this case, the fall in blood pressure is accompanied by a fall in vascular resistance to beneath the pretreatment level, and stroke volume also returns to normal.

Metabolic effects

Regulation of extracellular potassium

Spontaneous hypokalaemia down to levels of approximately 2·5 mmol/l is found to occur in approximately 50% of all patients admitted to hospital with acute severe pathology. These include patients with myocardial infarction, cerebrovascular accident, hypothermia, multiple injuries and febrile diseases (16). After institution of treatment of the underlying disease, this hypokalaemia disappears spontaneously in the course of a few days. Oral administration of extra potassium does not influence this course.

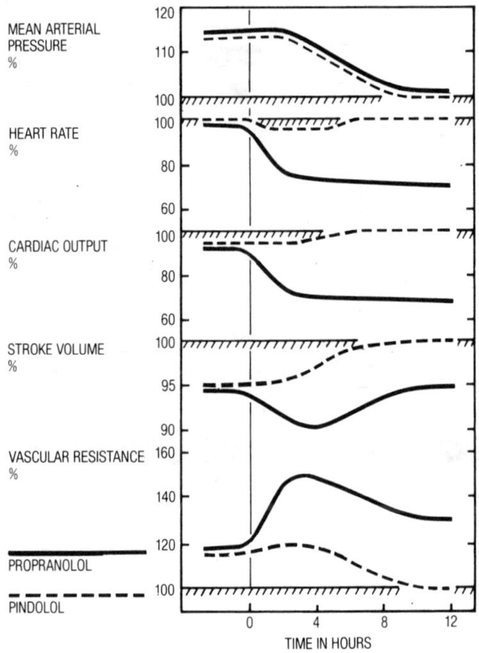

Figure 10. Time course of haemodynamic changes during treatment of hypertension with a β-blocker devoid of ISA (propranolol) and a β-blocker with strong ISA (pindolol). The dashed-lines (100%) indicate the haemodynamic status in normotensive subjects.

More insight into the background of this stress-induced hypokalaemia is provided by the work of Struthers *et al.* (17). Under the influence of infusion of a relatively small dose of adrenaline, plasma potassium decreases by 0·6–0·8 mmol/l within 15–30 min. Pretreatment with thiazide diuretics potentiates this hypokalaemia. The adrenaline infusion resulted in a rise of the plasma adrenaline to levels of approximately 700 pg/ml. Similar values have also been reported in the above-named patients with acute pathological conditions. Possibly, therefore, adrenaline is the link between stress and hypokalaemia.

Vincent *et al.* studied the question whether β-receptor stimulation may be held responsible for this phenomenon (18–20). Infusion of the $\beta_1+\beta_2$-agonist, isoprenaline, is followed by a dose-dependent decrease of plasma potassium by 0·6–0·8 mmol/l with an increase of heart rate of 40–50 beats/min. This hypokalaemic effect cannot be prevented by treatment with the β_1-selective blocker atenolol, but it can be prevented by pretreatment with the non-selective blocker propranolol. Apparently, stimulation of a β_2-receptor is responsible for the hypokalaemia. Since adrenaline is the natural β_2-agonist, this is in agreement with the findings of Struthers *et al.* The fall of the plasma potassium occurs so rapidly (15–30 min), that renal excretion of potassium cannot be held responsible for it. An alternative explanation is uptake of extracellular potassium by the cells. The body's largest store of potassium is localized in the skeletal muscles. Striated muscle cells possess β_2-receptors on their surface. Activation of these receptors stimulates the enzyme Na-K-AtPase, as the result of which more potassium is pumped into the cell and the extracellular potassium level decreases. Isoprenaline is found to raise plasma noradrenaline, also by stimulation of a β_2-receptor. A possible mechanism is an increased release of noradrenaline from the postganglionic sympathetic nerve fibres, by way of stimulation of presynaptic β_2-receptors (20).

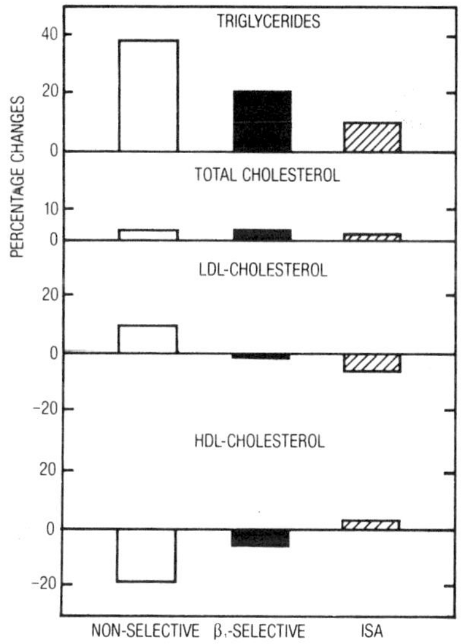

Figure 11. Effects of β-blockers on plasma lipids (21).

Lipid metabolism

As appears from a study of the literature by Van Brummelen, β-blockers without ISA cause a rise of the plasma triglycerides and a decrease of the high density lipoprotein (HDL)/low density lipoprotein (LDL)-cholesterol ratio (21). With β_1-selective blockers, these effects are much less pronounced. β-Blockers with ISA, however, not affect the plasma triglyceride level and cause an increase of the HDL/LDL-cholesterol ratio (Fig. 11).

Pathophysiological considerations

β_1-Selective blockers are found not to block 'stress hypokalaemia'. The same holds true for the release of noradrenaline that is increased under these circumstances. In hypertension, β-blockers are prescribed for purposes of 'prevention', i.e. inter alia for the prevention of the lethal complications of myocardial infarction. The blockade of the β_2-receptor by non-selective β-blockers, which prevents the release of noradrenaline and the occurrence of hypokalaemia, might well play an important part in the cardioprotective effect of β-blockers. A situation in acute myocardial infarction with high noradrenaline levels and a low plasma potassium, is precisely the condition where cardiac arrhythmias are to be feared most.

Arrhythmias are the main cause of early death in acute myocardial infarction. It is clear that blockade of β_2-receptors, both presynaptic and those on striated muscle cells, may be useful in this respect. Adrenaline potentiates the hypokalaemia induced by thiazide diuretics. This will make it clear that the combination of a selective β-blocker with a thiazide diuretic in the same tablet may be a scary experiment.

Just as the level of blood pressure, the magnitude of the HDL/LDL-cholesterol ratio is an indicator of the risk of cardiovascular disease. The lower this ratio, the higher the risk of cardiovascular complications. Accordingly, it would appear to be obvious that in the treatment of hypertension an attempt should be made to raise the HDL/LDL-cholesterol ratio. However, there is as yet no scientific proof of the assumption that 'spontaneous' changes in the lipid metabolism have the same significance as drug-induced effects.

Side-effects

The lung

Selective blockers are alleged to be safer in patients suffering from or predisposed to obstructive airways diseases. Since the major airways (trachea and main bronchi) also contain β_1-receptors, even highly β_1-selective blockers are not absolutely safe in these patients. If such patients require antihypertensive medication, plenty of alternatives are available nowadays. Also, with increasing dosage the selectivity of most β-blockers decreases rapidly. This does not alter the fact that for patients with a chronic obstructive lung disease, who require simultaneous treatment with a β_2-mimetic agent, a β_1-selective blocker is to be preferred.

Diabetes mellitus

Frequently, the administration of β-blockers to diabetics is quite permissible (22,23). However, it has been found that during an insulin-induced hypoglycaemia in these patients, non-selective β-blockade prolongs the duration of hypoglycaemia (24,25), in contrast to β_1-selective β-blockers or β-blockers with ISA (26,27). A potential danger of selective β-blockers in patients with diabetes mellitus is precisely the hypoglycaemia that occasionally occurs after all. This is the strongest stimulus conceivable to the adrenal glands to release adrenaline. The above-named hypokalaemia that results from this, definitely constitutes a threat to the patient with diabetes mellitus who in any case runs an increased risk of atherosclerosis and the concomitant cardiac complications. Accordingly, in patients with diabetes mellitus, the non-selective ISA β-blocker appears to offer advantages rather than disadvantages.

Bradycardia, cardiac failure, disorders of the peripheral blood circulation

Excessive bradycardia, cardiac decompensation (failure) and disorders of the peripheral circulation may be a direct consequence of the negative inotropic and chronotropic effects that derive from cardiac β-blockade. It has occasionally been suggested that β_1-selective blockers would give rise less frequently to disorders of the peripheral circulation and/or Raynaud phenomena because they do not block the vascular β_2-receptors. This, however, is definitely not correct, as also appears from the above-named haemodynamic effects of selective and non-selective β-blockers without ISA. Presence of sufficient ISA is found to be of far greater importance in this connection, irrespective of the presence or absence of β_1-receptor selectivity.

Apparently, the main element is not the blockade of the vascular β_2-receptor, but maintenance of peripheral perfusion (cardiac output). β-Blockers with sufficient ISA maintain the peripheral perfusion and cause no vasoconstriction (28). Excessive bradycardia occurs less often with β-blockers with a substantial degree of ISA (29). The significantly weaker negative inotropic effect of β-blockers with a substantial amount of ISA does not mean, however, that these drugs might safely be prescribed for patients with clinically manifest cardiac failure. In these patients, the sympathetic tone and the plasma noradrenaline level are raised, so that in them any β-blocker acts as an antagonist and will only cause further deterioration of the clinical condition.

The β-blocker withdrawal syndrome

When chronic β-blockade is discontinued suddenly, the β-blocker withdrawal syndrome may occur (30,31). In patients with ischaemic heart diseases, this syndrome may manifest itself as severe angina pectoris or impending myocardial infarction. Sudden cardiac death has also been described. In patients with uncomplicated hypertension, the syndrome runs a less dramatic course and manifests itself for a few days as restlessness, palpitations, disorders of sleep, tachycardia and rebound or overshoot hypertension. The syndrome is tentatively attributed to an increased number of β-receptors ('up-regulation'), secondary to the β-blockade, resulting in 'hypersensitivity' to sympathetic stimulation (30). It is important to note that the β-blocker withdrawal syndrome does not occur after discontinuation of the administration of β-blockers with a substantial degree of ISA. It has been reported, in fact, that during treatment with these agents there is no 'up-regulation' but, on the contrary, a 'down-regulation' of the number of β-receptors.

Effects on the central nervous system

Vivid dreams, disorders of sleep, depression, hallucinations and problems with concentration are interpreted as effects of β-blocking drugs on the central nervous system. Most β-blockers are more or less lipophilic and consequently can easily penetrate through the blood–brain barrier from the blood. There are increasingly convincing indications that hydrophilic β-blockers cause fewer central side-effects (32–34) as should be expected on physicochemical grounds. If these symptoms occur during treatment with a lipophilic β-blocker, switching to a hydrophilic β-blocker may provide a solution.

Conclusions

Although pharmacologically different in many respects, all β-blockers are equally effective where their action on blood pressure is concerned. However, depending on such properties as ISA, β_1-selectivity and lipophilicity, they differ in their haemodynamic profiles, their effects of lipid and potassium metabolism and their side-effects. Whether these differences between the various β-blockers result also in different effects on the increased cardiovascular risk that is associated with hypertension is still an open question. However, sound knowledge of the various properties of the different β-blockers will lead in practice to a discriminating and critical use of these agents. In this way, the balance of efficacy, safety and tolerability of these drugs can be optimized for the individual patient. Ultimately, this may result in better compliance and consequently, in a better prognosis.

References

(1) Black JW, Stephenson JS. Pharmacology of a new adrenergic β-receptor blocking compound (Nethalide). *Lancet* 1962; **ii**: 311–314.
(2) Prichard BNC. Hypotensive action of pronethalol. *Br Med J* 1964; **1**: 1227–1228.
(3) Memorandum from a WHO/ISH Meeting. Guidelines for the treatment of mild hypertension. *Hypertension* 1983; **5**: 394–397.
(4) Prichard BNC. Beta-adrenergic receptor blockade in hypertension; past, present and future. *Br J Clin Pharmac* 1978; **5**: 379–399.
(5) Cruickshank JM. The clinical importance of cardio-selectivity and lipophilicity in β-blockers. *Am Heart J* 1980; **100** (2): 160–178.
(6) Reale A, Motolese M. Partial agonist activity of β-adrenergic blocking agents and cardiac performance: a review. *Eur Heart J* 1981; **2**: 245–251.
(7) Kendall MJ. Are selective β-adrenoceptor blocking drugs an advantage? *J Roy Coll Phys London* 1981; **15**: 33–40.
(8) Loris WJ, Taylor H, McNeil JJ, Jarrott B, Rand MJ. Clinical pharmacology of adrenergic adrenoceptor-blocking drugs. *Am Heart J* 1982; **104**: 407–412.
(9) Thadani U. Beta blockers in hypertension. *Am J Cardiol.* 1983; **52**: 10D–15D.
(10) McDevitt DG. β-Adrenoceptor blocking drugs and partial agonist activity; it is clinically relevant? *Drugs* 1983; **25**: 331–338.
(11) Taylor SH. Intrinsic sympathomimetic activity: clinical fact or fiction? *Am J. Cardiol* 1983; **52**: 16D–26D.
(12) Breckenridge A. Which beta blocker? *Br Med J* 1983; **286**: 1085–1088.
(13) Man in 't Veld AJ, Schalekamp MADH. Effects of 10 different β-adrenoceptor antagonists on hemodynamics, plasma renin activity, and plasma norepinephrine in hypertension: the key role of vascular resistance changes in relation to partial agonist activity. *J Cardiovasc Pharmac* 1983; **5** (suppl 2): S30–S45.
(14) Man in 't Veld AJ, Schalekamp MADH. Haemodynamic consequences of intrinsic sympathomimetic activity and cardioselectivity in β-blocker therapy for hypertension. *Eur Heart J* 1983; **4**(suppl. D): 31–41.
(15) Man in 't Veld AJ, Schalekamp MADH. How intrinsic sympathomimetic activity modulates the haemodynamic responses to β-adrenoceptor antagonists. A clue to the nature of their antihypertensive mechanism. *Br J Clin Pharmac* 1982; **13**(suppl. 2): 245S–259S.
(16) Morgan DB, Young RM. Acute transient hypokalaemia: new interpretation of a common event. *Lancet* 1982; **ii**: 751–752.
(17) Struthers AD, Whitesmith R, Reid JL. Prior thiazide diuretic treatment increases adrenaline-induced hypokalemia. *Lancet* 1983; **i**: 1358–1360.
(18) Vincent HH, Man in 't Veld AJ, Boomsma F, Derkx FHM, Wenting GJ, Schalekamp MADH. Cardioprotection by blockade of β_2-adrenoceptors. *Eur Heart J* 1983; **4**(suppl. D): 109–115.
(19) Vincent HH, Boomsma F, Man in 't Veld AJ, Derkx FHM, Wenting GJ, Schalekamp MADH. Effects of selective and non-selective β-agonists on plasma potassium and norepinephrine. *J Cardiovasc Pharmac* 1984; **6**: 107–114.
(20) Vincent HH, Man in 't Veld AJ, Boomsma F, Wenting GJ, Schalekamp MADH. Elevated plasma noradrenaline levels in response to β-adrenoceptor stimulation. *Br J Clin Pharmac* 1982; **13**: 717–721.

(21) Van Brummelen P. The relevance of intrinsic sympathomimetic activity for β-blocker-induced changes in plasma lipids. *J Cardiovasc Pharmac* 1983; **5**(suppl. 1):S51–55.

(22) Barrett AH, Leslie D, Watkins PJ. Can insulin-treated diabetics be given β-adrenergic blocking drugs? *Br Med J* 1980; **280**: 976–977.

(23) Fitzgerald JD. Effects of propranolol on blood sugar, insulin and free fatty acids. *Diabetalogia* 1968; **5**: 339–341.

(24) Bolli G, De Feo P, Campagnucci P, Cartechini MG, Angeletti G, Santeusanio F, Brunetti P. Important role of adrenergic mechanisms in acute, glucose comter-regulation following insulin-induced hypoglycemia in Type I diabetes. *Diabetes* 1982; **32**: 641–647.

(25) Deacon SP, Karunanayake A, Barrett D. Acebutolol, atenolol and propranolol and metabolic responses to acute hypoglycaemia in diabetics. *Br Med J* 1977; **2**: 1255–1257.

(26) Raptis S, Rosenthal J, Welzel D, Moulopoulos S. Effects of cardioselective and non-cardioselective β-blockade on adrenaline-induced metabolic and cardiovascular responses in man. *Eur J Clin Pharmac* 1981; **2D**: 17–22.

(27) Schlütter KJ, Aellig WH, Petersen KG, Riebaud HC, Welirli A, Kerp L. The influence of β-adrenoceptor drugs with and without intrinsic sympathomimetic activity on the hormonal responses to hypo- and hyper-glycaemia. *Br J Clin Pharmac* 1982; **13**(suppl 2): 407S–417S.

(28) Man in 't Veld AJ, Schalekamp MADH. Hemodynamics of β-blockers. In: Kostis, De Felice eds, New York: Raven Press, 1984: 229–251.

(29) Aellig WH. Pindolol—a β-adrenoceptor blocking drug with partial agonist activity: clinical pharmacological consideration. *Br J Clin Pharmac* 1982; **13**(suppl 2): 187S–192S.

(30) Prichard BNC, Walden RJ. The syndrome associated with the withdrawal of β-adrenergic receptor blocking drugs. *Br J Clin Pharmac* 1982; **13**(suppl 2): 337S–344S.

(31) Rangno RE, Langlois S. Comparison of withdrawal phenomenon after propranolol. *Br J Clin Pharmac* 1982; **13**(suppl 2): 345S–352S.

(32) Betts TA, Alford C. Beta-blocking drugs and sleep. A controlled diet. *Drugs* 1983; **25**(suppl 2): 268–272.

(33) Cave-Smith R, Kirk CA. New Drugs: β blockers and sympathomimetics. *Br Med J* 1983; **286**: 1650–1651.

(34) Westerlund A. A comparison of the central nervous system side effects caused by lipophilic and hydrophilic β-blockers. *Drugs* 1983; **25**(suppl 2): 280–281.

Acute and long-term haemodynamic effects of bopindolol

A. H. VAN DEN MEIRACKER, A. J. MAN IN 'T VELD and M. A. D. H. SCHALEKAMP

Department of Internal Medicine I, University Hospital Dijkzigt, Erasmus University, Rotterdam

Summary

The haemodynamic effects of the first dose of bopindolol, 2 mg, was monitored invasively for 24 h in ten patients with uncomplicated essential hypertension. The haemodynamic studies were repeated, after the patients had been treated with bopindolol, 2 mg once daily, for 3 weeks. Isoprenaline was infused 24 h after the first dose of bopindolol and 1 week after withdrawal from chronic treatment, in order to assess the degree of cardiac and vascular β-adrenoceptor blockade. Before treatment baseline values of mean arterial pressure (MAP), heart rate (HR), cardiac output (CO) and total peripheral resistance (TPR) were 124 ± 3 (mean ± SEM) mmHg, 67 ± 3 beats/min, 5·1 ± 0·2 l/min and 1990 ± 126 dyn/s/cm^{-5} respectively. The maximal effects on HR and CO were seen within 2 h after administration of bopindolol: HR and CO decreased by 11·6 ± 1·1 ($p<0\cdot001$) and 11·9 ± 3·1% ($p<0\cdot01$) respectively. The reduction in CO was associated with a rise in TPR of 11·6 ± 4·6% ($p<0\cdot05$). Mean arterial blood pressure did not change within 4 h after dosing, but it had decreased by 9·9 ± 1·8% ($p<0\cdot001$) after 24 h. At that time changes in HR (0·2 ± 2,6%), CO (3·0 ± 3·7%) and TPR (−9,2 ± 4·1%) were not significantly different from baseline. After 3 weeks of treatment MAP was lowered by 8·5 ± 2·2% ($p<0\cdot01$). This was associated with a decrease in HR of 17·7 ± 4·0% ($p<0\cdot01$), but not with significant changes in CO (−10·3 ± 6·0%) or TPR (6·8 ± 8·2%). The isoprenaline infusion studies yielded a shift of the HR-dose-response curve to the right by a dose-factor of 12·7 24 h after the first dose of bopindolol, whereas the fall in diastolic pressure during isoprenaline was completely blunted. One week after stopping bopindolol, the HR-dose-response curve was still shifted to the right by a dose-factor of 2·2, and the fall in diastolic pressure during isoprenaline was still blunted. Despite significant β-blockade one week after discontinuation of bopindolol, MAP (−3·7 ± 2·2%) and HR (1·8 ± 5·4%) were not different from pretreatment values. Our findings indicate, that bopindolol is a potent non-selective β-blocker with

The position of bopindolol, a new β-blocker, edited by P. A. van Zwieten, 1987: Royal Society of Medicine Services International Congress and Symposium Series No. 106, published by Royal Society of Medicine Services Limited.

with a long duration of action. The drug does not seem to possess a significant degree of partial agonist activity.

Introduction

Bopindolol is a new non-selective β-adrenoceptor antagonist. It is a prodrug, which first has to be hydrolysed into an active metabolite before it exert its β-adrenoceptor blocking activity (1). Studies in healthy volunteers have shown that on a weight basis bopindolol is ten times as potent as pindolol in antagonizing exercise or isoprenaline-induced tachycardia (2). Besides this relatively high potency the drug also has a long duration of action, which makes it suitable for once daily or even less frequent administration (3). Limited experimental and clinical evidence indicates that bopindolol possesses a mild degree of intrinsic sympathomimetic activity (ISA) (4,5). Detailed haemodynamic studies on the onset and maintenance of the antihypertensive action of bopindolol are not available. Therefore we studied the acute and long-term haemodynamic effects of bopindolol in ten patients with uncomplicated essential hypertension.

Patients and methods

Ten male patients with mild to moderate essential hypertension were recruited from the out-pateint hypertension clinic. Their mean age was 48 years (range 36–60 years). When untreated, all patients had diastolic blood pressures of 95 mmHg or higher on at least three different occasions in the out-patient clinic. Secondary forms of hypertension were excluded by clinical and laboratory evaluation, including isotope renography. None of the patients had evidence for ischaemic heart disease, cerebrovascular disease or chronic obstructive lung disease.

Values of serum creatinine, blood urea nitrogen and electrolytes were all within the normal range of the laboratory. The purpose and procedures of the study were explained to the patients, who all gave their consent to participate. The study protocol was approved by the Local Hospital Ethical Review Committee.

Study protocol

The study was designed as a single blind placebo controlled trial. It was divided in two parts: an acute in-patient study for 24 h and a chronic out-patient study lasting for 7 weeks. Antihypertensive medication, if any, was discontinued at least 3 weeks before the study was started. After this washout-period placebo capsules, once daily, were provided during the first 3 weeks. At the end of the second week of this placebo period the patients were admitted to the hospital in order to study invasively the acute haemodynamic effects of bopindolol, 2 mg. After an overnight bedrest recumbent haemodynamic measurements were started 1–2 h after arterial and venous catheterizations. When stable baseline haemodynamic values were obtained for 2 h the first dose of bopindolol, 2 mg orally, was given. Systemic arterial pressure and heart rate were monitored continuously. Cardiac output was measured at hourly intervals. The measurements were interrupted from 23 h 00 to 07 h 00. At the end of the acute study blockade of cardiac and vascular β-adrenoceptors was assessed by isoprenaline infusion. The results of this isoprenaline infusion were compared to those obtained during placebo 1 week before. After the acute study the patients went back on placebo and they were seen in the out-patient clinic at weekly intervals in order to study non-invasively the chronic haemodynamic effects of bopindolol. During each visit supine blood pressure and heart rate were measured between 08 h 00 and 10 h 00. During weeks 4, 5 and 6 the dose of bopindolol was adjusted weekly from 1 to 2, and to 4 mg once daily depending on the blood pressure response (diastolic pressure < 90 mmHg). At the end of the sixth week, supine resting cardiac output was measured non-invasively. At that time the dose of bopindolol was $2 \cdot 6 \pm 0 \cdot 4$ mg (mean ± SEM). After the sixth week the patients were switched to placebo and one week later isoprenaline infusions were repeated.

Invasive haemodynamic measurements

Arterial pressure was measured in the brachial artery of the non-dominant arm, which was cannulated with a 1·0 mm diameter teflon catheter (Plastimed, Saint-Leu-la-Forêt, France) by means of the Seldinger technique. For measurements of cardiac output a flow directed Swan Ganz thermodilution catheter was introduced percutaneously into an antecubital vein. Cardiac output was determined in triplicate by bolus injections of 10 ml of ice-cold dextrose 5%. Total peripheral vascular resistance (TPR) was calculated as TPR = 80X(MAP-RAP)/CO, where MAP = mean arterial pressure, RAP = mean right atrial pressure and CO = cardiac output.

Non-invasive haemodynamic measurements

Supine blood pressure and heart rate were measured every 5 min for 1 h by an automatic oscillometric device (Datascope, Accutorr I, Datascope Corp, Paramus, USA). The values of blood pressure and heart rate obtained during 1 h were averaged. Supine cardiac output was measured by an isotope dilution technique at the end of the blood pressure measurements (6). 99 m-Technetium labelled human serum albumin (Technescan HSA, Mallinckrodt Diagnostica BV, Petten, The Netherlands), 100–200 μCi, was used as the indicator. After rapid intravenous injection of the isotope, time-concentration curves were recorded for 2 min by precordial counting of the radioactivity using a single probe. Additional recordings were made after 5 and 10 min, when blood was sampled for counting radioactivity. Cardiac output was calculated by means of the Steward Hamilton formula. TPR was calculated as 80XMAP/CO.

Isoprenaline infusions

Isoprenaline was infused through an indwelling cannula in a forearm vein. The heart rate during the infusions was derived from a continuous recorded ECG, and arterial pressure was measured directly in a brachial or radial artery. After baseline values of heart rate and systemic arterial pressure were obtained during continuous infusion of saline (2 ml/min) for 20 min, the infusion was switched to isoprenaline. The doses of isoprenaline during placebo and 1 week after withdrawal were 3·5, 7, 14, 35 and 70 ng/kg/min. At the end of the acute study the doses were 35, 70, 140, 350 and 700 ng/kg/min. The dose of isoprenaline was increased every 10 min until a rise in heart rate of 25 beats/min was obtained. The average value of heart rate in the last 2 min of each dose step was used to construct heart rate log-dose-response curves. In every patient the dose of isoprenaline to increase the heart rate by 25 beats/min (CD25) was calculated.

Statistics

Data are presented as means ± SEM. Haemodynamic parameters relevant to body size were corrected for 1·73 m^2 body surface area. For comparison Student's two tailed *t*-test for paired observations was used: *p*-values $<0{\cdot}05$ were considered to indicate a significant difference.

Results

Acute haemodynamic effects

Averaged baseline values of MAP, HR, CO and TPR 1–2 h prior to the first dose of bopindolol were 124 ± 3 mmHg, 67 ± 3 beats/min, 5·1 ± 0·2 l/min and 1990 ± 126 dynes/s/cm^{-5}, respectively. Within 2 h after administration of bopindolol maximal effects on HR and CO were observed. At that time HR was reduced to 61 ± 2 beats/min ($p<0{\cdot}001$) and CO had decreased to 4·5 ± 0·2 l/min ($p<0{\cdot}01$), (Fig. 1). The fall in CO was associated with a rise in TPR to 2161 ± 128 dynes/s/cm^{-5} ($p<0{\cdot}01$). In contrast to the changes in HR, CO and TPR, MAP did not change within 4 h after dosing: 5 h after dosing MAP had fallen to 113 ± 4 mmHg ($p<0{\cdot}01$). This decrease in MAP was associated with return of TPR and CO towards baseline values. At the end of the acute study MAP was lowered to 112 ± 2 mmHg (−9·9%, $p<0{\cdot}001$). By that time HR (68 ± 2 beats/min, +0·2%), CO (5·2 ± 0·2 l/min, +3·0%) and TPR (1694 ± 73 dynes/s/cm^{-5}, −9·2%) were not different from baseline values.

Long-term haemodynamic effects

The respective values of MAP, HR, CO and TPR during placebo were 119 ± 3 mmHg, 75 ± 3 beats/min, 5·6 ± 0·5 l/min and 1813 ± 144 dynes/s/cm^{-5}. After treatment for 3 weeks MAP was decreased to 109 ± 4 mmHg (−8·5 ± 2·2%, $p<0{\cdot}01$). This fall in MAP was associated with a reduction of HR to 61 ± 2 beats/min (−17·7 ± 4·0%, $p<0{\cdot}01$). No significant changes in CO or TPR were observed. The values of CO and TPR at the end of the chronic treatment period were 4·9 ± 0·3 l/min (−10·3 ± 6·0%) and 1863 ± 82 dynes/s/cm^{-5} (+6·8 ± 8·2%) respectively. One week after withdrawal of bopindolol, MAP (115 ± 4 mmHg) and HR (71 ± 3 beats/min) were not different from the values of these parameters during the initial placebo period.

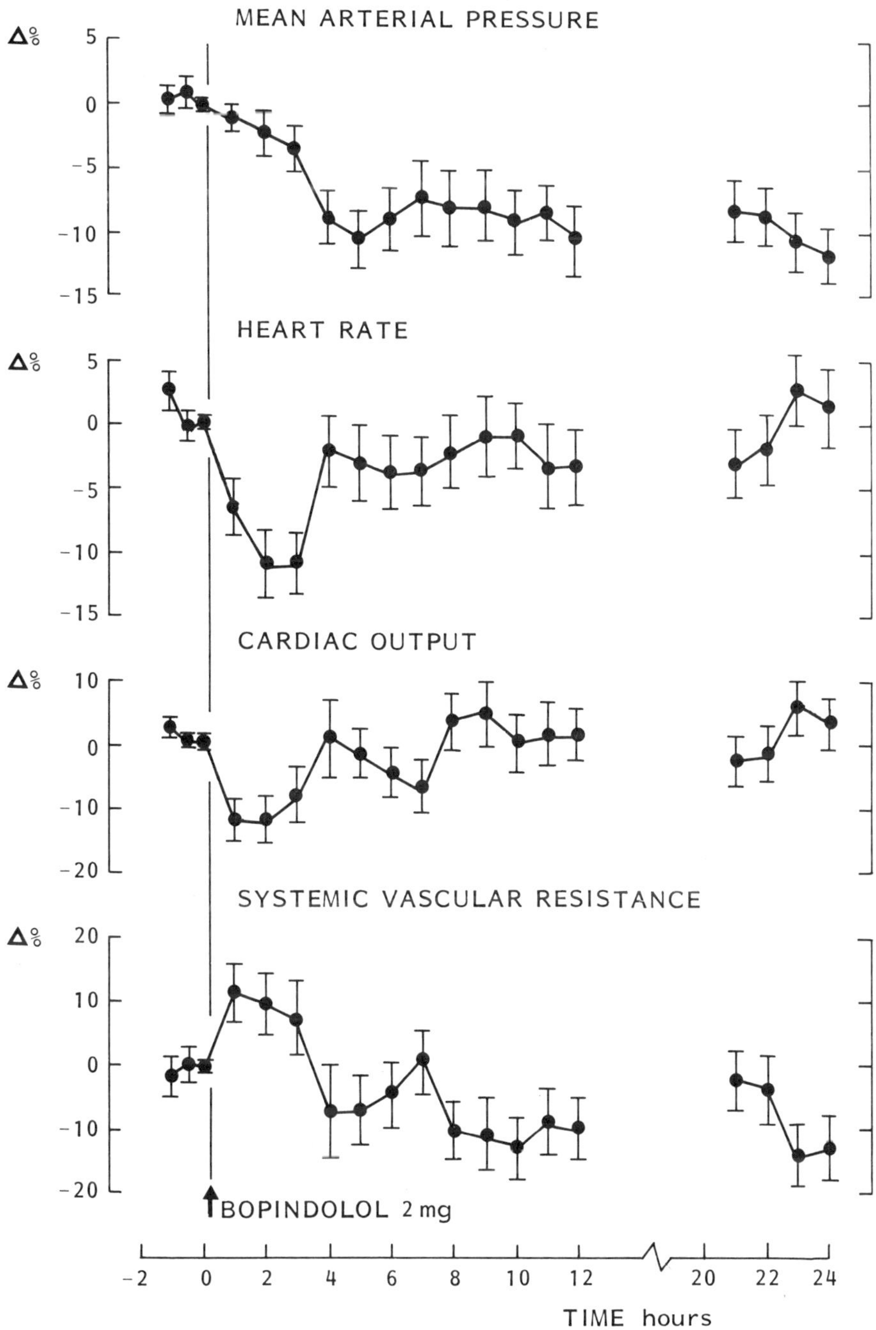

Figure 1. Time course of changes in mean arterial pressure, heart rate, cardiac output and systemic vascular resistance after the first oral dose of bopindolol, 2 mg.

Isoprenaline infusion studies

The CD25 during placebo was 21 ± 3 ng/kg/min. The CD25 was increased to 265 ± 55 ng/kg/min 24 h after the first dose of bopindolol, 2 mg. Despite this much higher dose of isoprenaline the fall in diastolic arterial pressure during isoprenaline infusion was abolished. One week after withdrawal from chronic treatment the CD25 was still elevated (51 ± 9 ng/kg/min, $p < 0{\cdot}01$), and the fall in diastolic arterial pressure during isoprenaline was still fully suppressed.

Discussion

The present study confirms earlier observations that monotherapy with bopindolol once daily is efficacious in lowering blood pressure for 24 h (3,7). Although bopindolol is a prodrug, studies in healthy volunteers have shown that blockade of cardiac as well as juxtaglomerular β-adrenoceptors is apparent within 2 h after an oral dose (8). The present observation, that a maximum effect on heart rate and cardiac output was seen 2 h after the first dose of bopindolol, is in agreement with these findings. Despite the rapid fall in cardiac output after bopindolol arterial pressure remained initially unchanged because of a transient increase of total peripheral vascular resistance. A significant fall in arterial pressure, which was due to return of total peripheral vascular resistance towards baseline values, was not seen until 5 h after dosing. The time course of haemodynamic changes after bopindolol is similar to the time course of haemodynamic changes after atenolol or timolol, two β-adrenoceptor blocking drugs lacking ISA (9,10).

Also, the long-term haemodynamic effects of bopindolol do not suggest that the drug has a pronounced degree of ISA. First, as reported in several other studies (3,7,11), basal heart rate was markedly reduced. Second, the maintenance of the antihypertensive effect was not associated with a fall in total peripheral vascular resistance. This haemodynamic profile contrasts with β-adrenoceptor antagonists with considerable ISA. These drugs, lower arterial pressure through reduction of total peripheral vascular resistance without major changes in cardiac output and heart rate, at least under basal conditions (12–14).

The extremely high β-adrenoceptor blocking potency of bopindolol and its long duration of action are confirmed by the results of the isoprenaline infusion studies. The heart rate-dose-response curve was shifted to the right by a dose-factor of nearly 13 24 h after the first dose of bopindolol, 2 mg. Moreover, 1 week after withdrawal from chronic treatment significant blockade of cardiac and vascular β-adrenoceptors was still present. Interestingly, despite blockade of β-adrenoceptors blood pressure was no longer significantly reduced. This finding therefore supports earlier suggestions, that a certain critical level of blockade of β-adrenoceptors is required for the full antihypertensive action of β-adrenoceptor blocking drugs (15).

In conclusion, bopindolol is a non-selective, potent, long-acting β-adrenoceptor antagonist, which can be administered once daily. From a haemodynamic point of view, the drug possesses little, if any, ISA in human hypertensives.

References

(1) Berthold R, Waite R, Weber H. Pharmacological studies with bopindolol: a new long-acting β-adrenoceptor antagonist. *Br J Pharmacol* 1981; **74**: 829P.

(2) Aellig WH. Pharmacological experiments in healthy volunteers with bopindolol, a long acting beta-adrenoceptor blocking drug with partial agonist activity. *Br J Clin Pharmac* 1985; **19**: 775–781.

(3) Andersson OK, Hedner T, Nyberg G. Acute and long-term antihypertensive effect of bopindolol. A non-selective beta-adrenergic blocker with ISA. *Europ J Clin Pharmacol* 1985; **29**: 281–285.

(4) Berthold R, Waite R, Weber H. Pharmacological studies with bopindolol: a new long-acting beta-adrenoceptor antagonist. *Br J Pharmac* 1981; **74**: 829.

(5) Nyberg G. Intrinsic sympathomimetic activity of bopindolol, a non-selective beta-adrenoceptor antagonist. *Br J Clin Pharmac* 1985; **20**: 242–243.

(6) Man in 't Veld AJ, Wenting GJ, Verhoeven RF, Schalekamp MADH. Quantitative radiocardiography by single probe counting using 99m technetium albumin. *Neth J Med* 1978; **21**: 166–175.

(7) Hulthen UL, van Brummelen P, Amann FW, Bühler FR. Antihypertensive efficacy of the new long-acting beta-blocker bopindolol as related to age. *J Cardiovasc Pharmacol* 1983; **5**: 426–429.

(8) Turner DR, Goodwin FJ, Knight AR, Littlejohns DW, Sharman VL, Vere DW. Bopindolol: a new long acting beta-receptor antagonist; its effects on haemodynamics, and on the renin response to tilting. *Br J Clinical Pharmacol* 1984; **17**: 295–299.

(9) Simon G, Franciosa JA, Gimenez HJ, Cohn JN. Short-term systemic hemodynamic adaptation to beta-adrenergic inhibition with atenolol in hypertensive patients. *Hypertension* 1981; **3**: 262–268.

(10) Colfer HT, Cottier C, Sanchez R, Julius S. Role of cardiac factors in the initial hypotensive action by beta-adrenoceptor blocking drugs. *Hypertension* 1984; **6**: 145–151.

(11) Van Brummelen P, Bolli P, Koolen MI, Staehelin HB, Bühler FR. Plasma lipid fractions during long-term monotherapy with the ISA-containing beta-adrenoceptor blocker bopindolol in hypertensive patients. *Br J Clin Pharmacol* 1984; **17**: 86–88.

(12) Man in 't Veld AJ, Schalekamp MADH. Effects of 10 different beta-adrenoceptor antagonists on hemodynamics, plasma renin activity, and plasma norepinephrine in hypertension: the key role of vascular resistance changes in relation to partial agonist activity. *J Cardiovasc Pharmacol* 1983; **5**(suppl 1): S30–45.

(13) Van den Meiracker A, Man in 't Veld AJ, Ritsema van Eck H, Wenting GJ, Schalekamp MADH. Direct 24-hour haemodynamic monitoring after starting beta-blocker therapy: studies with pindolol in hypertension. *J. Hypertension* 1984; **2**(suppl 3): 581–583.

(14) Van den Meiracker AH, Man in 't Veld AJ, Ritsema van Eck HJ, Schalekamp MADH. Systemic and renal vasodilatation after beta-adrenoceptor blockade with pindolol; a hemodynamic study on the onset and maintenance of its antihypertensive effect. *Am Heart J* 1986; **112**: 368–374.

(15) Korner PI. Beta-blockers, autoregulation and experimental design (Editorial). *Hypertension* 1984; **6**: 140–144.

Influence of bopindolol and atenolol on 24-hour cardiac frequency

P. FITSCHA, W. MEISNER and B. TISO

2nd Department of Internal Medicine (Heartstation), General Policlinic, Vienna, Austria

Summary

The effects of atenolol, a selective β-adrenoceptor blocker without intrinsic sympathomimetic activity (ISA) and bopindolol, a selective β-adrenoceptor blocker with ISA on circadian heart rate, was studied in ten patients with coronary heart disease ($n=4$) or hypertension ($n=6$). The patients were treated in a randomized cross-over study with single doses of 100 mg atenolol and 1 mg bopindolol.

Atenolol lowered the averaged circadian heart rate significantly ($p<0 \cdot 001$) from 70 to 59 beats/min. The rate decreased both during the day and at night. After bopindolol the average circadian heart rate decreased only slightly from 69 to 64 beats/min. The heart rate was reduced during the day but not during the night.

After atenolol nine out of ten patients developed hourly heart rates of less than 55 beats/min compared to three patients taking bopindolol. After atenolol there was a significant increase of hourly segments with a heart rate of <55 beats/min from 11 to 85 and also for hourly segments with a heart rate of <50 beats/min from 0 to 46 whereas no significant change could be detected when taking bopindolol.

Both drugs produced similar reductions in exercise-induced increases in heart rate and systolic blood pressure and these effects persisted for more than 24 h.

Introduction

Bopindolol is a new long-acting non-selective β-adrenoceptor antagonist (1). Animal pharmacological studies have indicated a mild membrane stabilizing effect and some intrinsic sympathomimetic activity (ISA) (2). Atenolol is a cardioselective β-adrenoceptor antagonist without intrinsic sympathomimetic activity (3,4).

It was the aim of our study to investigate the influence of both substances on 24-h cardiac frequency.

The position of bopindolol, a new β-blocker, edited by P. A. van Zwieten, 1987: Royal Society of Medicine Services International Congress and Symposium Series No. 106, published by Royal Society of Medicine Services Limited.

Method

After informed consent was obtained an in-patient study was carried out in a total of ten patients (three female, seven male) with an average age of 52 years (range 35–60 years), with the diagnoses: coronary heart disease ($n=4$) and hypertension ($n=6$). At day 1 (control) a commercially available Holter recorder (ICR) was applied at 08 h 00 to register the electrocardiogram in two leads for 48 h. At 08 h 00 the following day a bicycle exercise test was performed, with the patient in a sitting position, at a work load of 1 Watt/kg body weight during 6 min. Blood pressure was measured, according to the method of Riva Rocci, at rest and at the end of the exercise test. Heart rate was determined electrocardiographically. Immediately after the exercise test patients were randomly allocated to receive either 1 mg bopindolol or 100 mg atenolol orally. Three hours later (11 h 00) the exercise test was repeated. The next day (08 h 00) it was repeated again. After a drug free interval of 72 h the procedure was repeated with alternating medication. The well-known contraindications against β-adrenoceptor blockers were respected. During the study the patients did not receive any other therapy and special attention was paid to ensure that no tranquillizers or hypnotics were given.

The statistical comparisons were performed with the *t*-test for paired differences and patterns analysed according to Dixon-Mood. Correlation was calculated by means of linear regression analysis.

Results

Bopindolol significantly reduced ($p<0{\cdot}05$) the total number of heart beats in 24 h: 98 846 ± 8809 beats before, vs 92 712 ± 9586 beats after, therapy. A greater effect could be demonstrated for atenolol: 100 822 ± 7309 beats before, vs 84 751 ± 9169 ($p<0{\cdot}001$), the difference between the two substances being significant ($p<0{\cdot}05$). This means that the average heart rate within 24 h decreased after atenolol from 70 to 59 beats/min and after bopindolol from 69 to 64 beats/min.

Analysing the 24-h heart rate pattern (Figs 1,2,3) a reduction of heart rate after atenolol could be detected during the day (09 h 00 to 20 h 00) from 74 to 61 beats/min ($p<0{\cdot}001$) and at night (23 h 00 to 03 h 00) from 62 to 53 beats/min ($p<0{\cdot}001$). After bopindolol, during the day, heart rate decreased from 73 to 66 beats/min ($p<0{\cdot}01$). However, during the night, heart rate remained unchanged. Correspondingly the minimal average heart rate during the night was 43 beats/min after atenolol and 50 beats/min after bopindolol.

In all patients taken together there was a total of 85 hourly segments with average heart rates of less than 55 beats/min after atenolol (control — 11 segments, $p<0{\cdot}01$). These bradycardia segments occurred in nine out of the ten patients (control: three patients, $p<0{\cdot}01$). During bopindolol treatment there were three patients before and three patients after therapy with bradycardias less than 55 beats/min. The segments with heart rates less than 55 beats/min increased from 11 to 22 (NS). There were six patients in whom the average hourly heart rate was even below 50 beats/min in the atenolol group, whereas this was only the case in two patients after treatment with bopindolol.

Blood pressure and heart rate at rest and during exercise are shown in Fig. 4. At rest, both forms of treatment significantly reduced systolic and diastolic blood pressure for 24 h by approximately the same degree in both groups. Atenolol reduced the heart

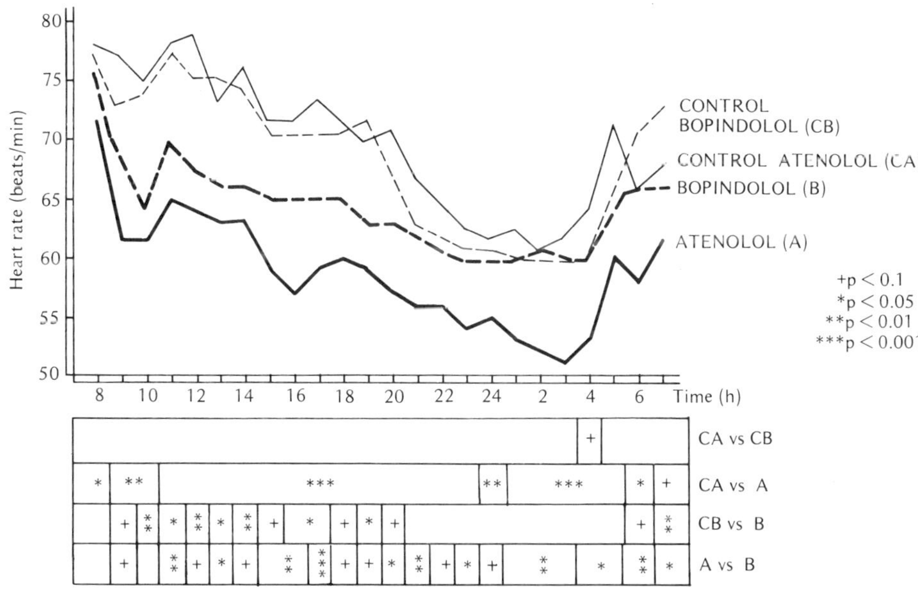

Figure 1. 24-h heart rate before and after bopindolol, compared with atenolol.

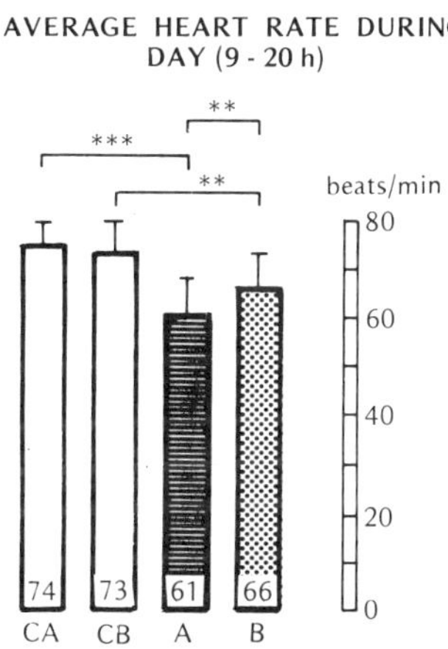

Figure 2. Average heart rate during daytime before (C) and after atenolol (A) or bopindolol (B).

rate at rest from 81 to 60 beats/min ($p<0\cdot001$) 3 h after intake. This effect lasted for 24 h, but was not so marked at the final test period (66 beats/min). There was no significant influence upon resting heart rate in the bopindolol treated patients. During exercise both β-adrenoceptor blockers caused almost the same significant reduction in the increase of systolic blood pressure and heart rate during 24 h. Thus we may assume that the doses of both drugs used were pharmacodynamically equieffective.

Discussion

In our study of circadian heart rate (Fig. 1) maximal heart rate was at about noon followed by a steady decline with lower values in the period between 01 h 00 and 04 h 00.

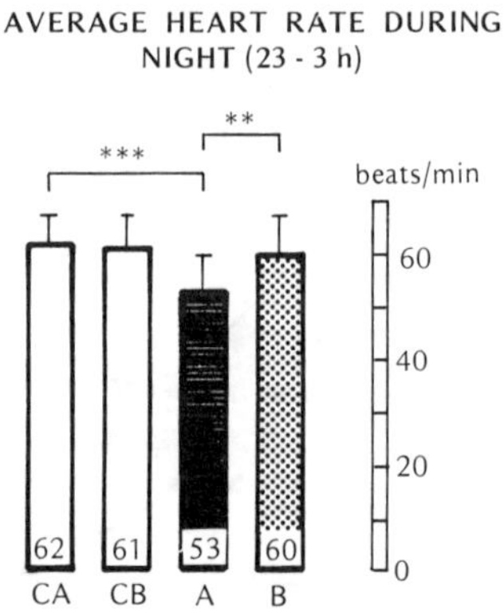

Figure 3. Average heart rate during night-time before (C) and after atenolol (A) or bopindolol (B).

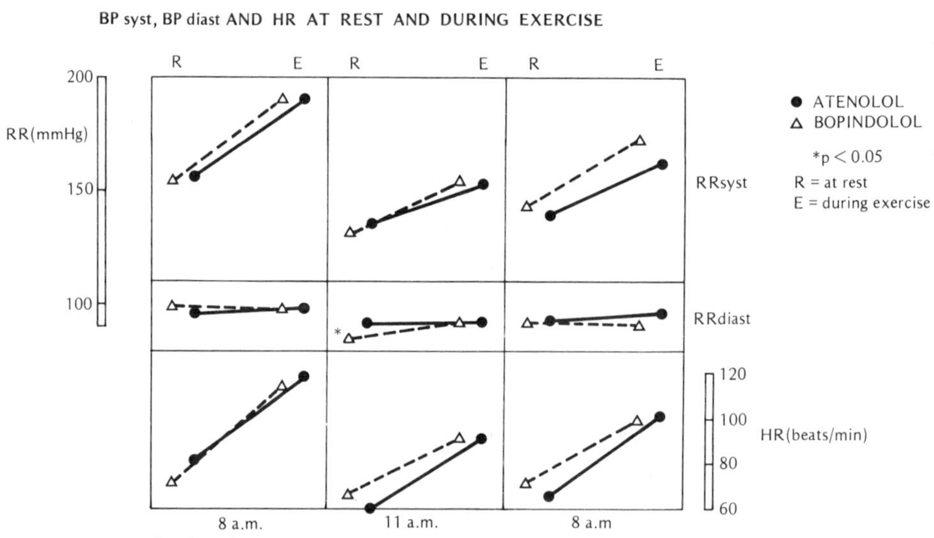

Figure 4. Systolic (BP syst.), diastolic (BP diast.) blood pressure and heart rate (HR) at rest (R) and during exercise (E) before and after bopindolol or atenolol.

In the morning (05 h 00) there was a significant increase in heart rate, which remained below the level at noon. The fall in heart rate during the night has already been described by others (5,6) and is assumed to be the result of a predominance of parasympathetic nervous activity during the night (7,8).

Atenolol lacking intrinsic sympathomimetic activity provoked a parallel shift of the heart rate (Fig. 1) towards lower values, i.e. produced a reduction in all the hourly segments of the recording. However, the effects of bopindolol were dependent on the prevailing state of sympathetic tone. During the night, when sympathetic tone is low, heart rate was not significantly influenced. During the daytime or during exercise (increased sympathetic tone) a significant reduction in heart rate could be detected. Probably, the reason for this pattern is a mild intrinsic sympathomimetic activity of bopindolol, since we have reported a slight increase of heart rate during night-time under pindolol which possesses high intrinsic sympathomimetic activity (9).

It is noteworthy that there were 46 hourly segments with an average heart rate less than 50 under atenolol, compared with five segments under bopindolol. Bopindolol is a long acting non-selective β-blocker which can be applied 'once a day' without causing unnecessary depression of heart rate.

References

(1) Aellig WH. Pharmacological experiments in healthy volunteers with bopindolol, a long-acting β-adrenoceptor blocking drug with partial agonist activity. *Br J Clin Pharmacol* 1985; **19**: 775–781.

(2) Berthold R, Waite R, Weber H. Pharmacological studies with bopindolol: a new long acting β-adrenoceptor antagonist. *Br J Pharmacol* 1981; **74**: 829P.

(3) Astrom H. Comparison of the effect on airway conductance of a new selective beta-adrenergic blocking drug, atenolol and propranolol in asthmatic subjects. *Scand J Resp Dis* 1975; **56**: 292–296.

(4) Conway FJ, Fitzgerald JD, McAinsh J, Rowlands DJ, Simpson WT. Human pharmacokinetic and pharmacodynamic studies on atenolol (ICI 66,082) a new cardioselective β-adrenoceptor blocking drug. *Br J Clin Pharmac* 1976; **3**: 267–272.

(5) Lown B, Tykocinski M, Garfein A, Brooks P. Sleep and ventricular premature beats. *Circulation* 1973; **48**: 691–701.

(6) Pickering ThG, Goulding L, Cobern BA. Diurnal variations in ventricular ectopic beats and heart rate. *Cardiovasc Med* 1977; **2**: 1013.

(7) Baust W, Bohnert B. The regulation of heart rate during sleep. *Exp Brain Res* 1966; **7**: 169–174.

(8) Samaan A. La fréquence cardiaque du chien en differentes conditions éxperimentals d'activities et de repos. *C R Soc Biol (Paris)* 1934; **115**: 1383–1388.

(9) Fitscha PB, Tiso B, Meisner W, Spitzer D. The effect of intrinsic sympathomimetic activity of β-adrenoceptor blockers on circadian heart rate. *Br J Clin Pharm* 1982; **13**: 211S–215S.

Pharmacokinetic and pharmacodynamic arguments for the explanation of the long action of bopindolol

J. GREVEL

University Department of Materia Medica, Stobhill General Hospital, Glasgow, UK

Summary

Bopindolol (BOP: a racemic mixture of the D and L isomer) is a prodrug which is rapidly metabolized *in vivo* into the β-adrenoceptor blocking compound hydrolysed bopindolol (HBOP). The half-life of the formation of HBOP was determined as 7·2 min after intravenous dosing. There is a close correlation between plasma levels of the drug measured specifically by high pressure liquid chromatography (HPLC) and by radioreceptor assay (RRA), indicating that HBOP is the only active compound in man. The elimination half-life of HBOP from plasma is about 4 h. After oral dosing of BOP the bioavailability of HBOP is about 70%.

As with many other β-adrenoceptor blockers there is a linear correlation between the reduction in exercise-induced heart rate, (REHR) and the logarithm of the plasma concentration of HBOP (C). The slope of this relationship is, however, exceptionally shallow. This means that a big drop in C is translated into only a small drop in REHR. Furthermore, HBOP is one of the most potent β-adrenoceptor blockers both *in vitro* and *in vivo* with a dissociation constant of about 0·1 nmol/1.

After a single oral dose of 1 mg BOP the peak effect (REHR = 20%) is reached after 3 h. Exercise heart rate is still 8·2% reduced 24 h after this dose. Predictions of effects (reduction in exercise-induced tachycardia), 24–72 h after multiple doses can be made using a one-compartment pharmacokinetic and a log-linear pharmacodynamic model. These predictions match well with experimental measurements thus proving that: HBOP is the only active metabolite; there is no deep kinetic compartment; and HBOP does not bind irreversibly to β-adrenergic receptors.

The position of bopindolol, a new β-blocker, edited by P. A. van Zwieten, 1987: Royal Society of Medicine Services International Congress and Symposium Series No. 106, published by Royal Society of Medicine Services Limited.

Pharmacokinetics

Bopindolol (BOP) is a prodrug which, after cleavage of a benzoyl ester bond, is transformed *in vivo* into the β-adrenoceptor blocking compound hydrolysed bopindolol (HBOP) (1). The rate of this metabolizing step was determined after giving intravenous doses of 1 mg BOP to healthy subjects. Under the assumption of a first order process a half-life of 7·2 min was estimated (2). After oral doses of 4 mg, HBOP appeared in plasma with a half-life of 0·84 h (2). This rate reflects both the absorption of BOP and the formation of HBOP. It was impossible, both after intravenous and oral dosing, to detect any unchanged BOP in plasma samples using a specific HPLC method (3). Results obtained by this analytical technique correlated 1 : 1 with measurements by a radioreceptor assay (RRA) on the basis of rat lung β_1 and β_2-receptors (3). This correlation indicated that HBOP is the only β-adrenoceptor blocking compound detectable in human plasma samples.

The temporal change of plasma concentrations of HBOP, C, is best described, after both intravenous and oral doses, by a one-compartment model where appearance and elimination of HBOP follows first order kinetics. An elimination half-life of HBOP in plasma ($t_{1/2}$) of about 4 h was determined by two groups of investigators using identical HPLC and RRA methods (2,3). This value does not change after repeated doses (3) and is comparable to those found for many other β-adrenoceptor blockers (4). Measurements of C after intravenous and oral dosing in the same healthy subjects were used to calculate the bioavailability (70%) and total clearance (0·3 l/kg/h) of HBOP (2).

Pharmacodynamics

The effective concentration in vivo

Any description or prediction of the time course of a drug effect *in vivo* needs an adequate model for the *in vivo* concentration-effect relationship. Which concentration is, however, eliciting the effect? For most β-adrenoceptor blockers it is apparently the plasma concentration itself. After single doses a defined plasma concentration in the ascending part of the pharmacokinetic profile is as potent as an equivalent concentration in the descending part of the curve. It is said that the plasma concentration is 'in phase' with the pharmacologic effect. A more detailed inspection of the available data reveals, however, that the maximum of the plasma concentration (C_{max}) with most β-adrenoceptor blockers is reached very early (~1 h) and that effect measurements are infrequent at time points before C_{max}.

In the case of oral doses of BOP C_{max} is not reached before 2 h. In a study by Aellig and co-workers (2) four exercise tests were performed within this time period and it was clearly demonstrated that the peak effect (REHR) was reached 1 h after C_{max}. It seems, therefore, that HBOP in plasma is not directly interacting with cardiac β-adrenoceptors. Indeed, the literature contains several reports on other β-adrenoceptor blockers which show the same phenomenon: practolol (5), labetalol (6), tertatolol (7). The following discussion of the concentration-effect relationship of bopindolol will not take this observation into account since the focus will be on the duration of effect and not on the time of the peak effect.

Isoproterenol dose ratio

The reduction in heart rate is generally used to assess the pharmacologic action of β-adrenoceptor blocking drugs in healthy volunteers. There is a physiologic (exercise) and pharmacologic (infusion of a β-adrenoceptor agonist) method to bring heart rate under adrenergic control.

Platzer and co-workers (3) measured the effect of oral BOP (2 mg) in healthy subjects under pharmacologic stimulation of heart rate as the isoproterenol dose ratio, DR:

$$DR = \frac{CD_{25} \text{ (antagonist present)}}{CD_{25} \text{ (antagonist absent)}}$$

where CD_{25} is the infusion rate of isoproterenol which increases heart rate by 25 beats/min. The relationship with the plasma concentration of HBOP, C, was established using the well-known Schild equation:

$$DR = (1/K_D) \times C + 1$$

where K_D is an apparent *in vivo* dissociation constant of HBOP for the β-adrenergic receptor. This equation shows that the effect of BOP measured as DR is linearly correlated with C: DR is therefore not the long-lasting effect of BOP and declines with the same half-life as C. The parameter K_D is a measure of the *in vivo* potency of BOP and interestingly lies in the same order of magnitude as the dissociation constant determined *in vitro* (0·1 nmol/1). The comparison with other β-adrenoceptor blocking drugs demonstrates that BOP is one of the most potent (3).

Reduction of exercise-induced heart rate

Physiologic stimulation of heart rate by exercise (bicycle ergometer) is reduced after BOP. The reduction in exercise-induced heart rate (REHR) and the reduction in exercise-induced tachycardia (REIT) (with resting heart rate subtracted) are expressed as a percentage compared to predose or placebo levels. It is known, ever since β-adrenoceptor blockers have been used in man, that both REHR and REIT decline linearly with time. Coltart and Shand (8) were the first to formulate the relationship with exponentially declining plasma concentrations:

$$\text{REHR, REIT} = \text{SLOPE} \times \log C + \text{INTERCEPT}$$

this equation was also established for BOP (3):

$$\text{REIT} = 10{\cdot}7 \times \log C + 6{\cdot}44$$

and is graphically depicted in Fig. 1. This log-linear relationship has its obvious limitations: at very high plasma concentrations there will be a maximal effect, E_{max}, which cannot be surpassed. Indeed, the log-linear relationship is a convenient linearization of the so-called E_{max} model:

$$\text{REHR, REIT} = \frac{E_{max} \times C}{IC_{50} + C}$$

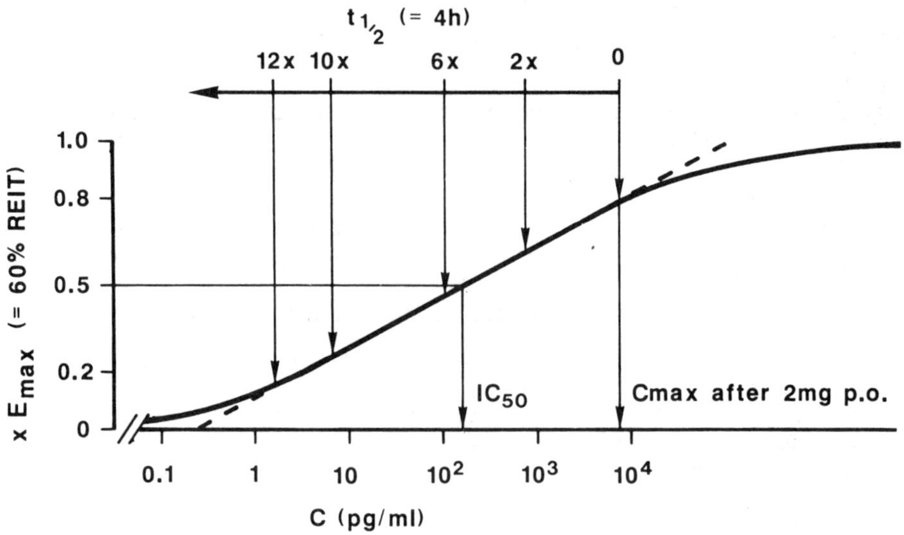

Figure 1. Relationship between the reduction in exercise-induced tachycardia, REIT, and the plasma concentration of HBOP, C, after a single oral dose of 2 mg BOP in a healthy volunteer. REIT on the ordinate is expressed as a fraction of E_{max} which itself is 60% (3). C is plotted logarithmically on the abscissa. The straight part of the curve is represented by the equation: $REIT = 10 \cdot 7 \times \log C + 6 \cdot 44$ (3). The entire curve reflects the assumption that the pharmacologic effect of HBOP (REIT) is a direct consequence of its binding to β-adrenoceptors according to the law of mass action. In this sense, the concentration which elicits $0 \cdot 5 \times E_{max}$ is the IC_{50} of HBOP. The temporal decline of the effect of BOP is illustrated on the upper horizontal axis. It starts at the right side with the highest REIT corresponding to C_{max} at $0 \times t_{1/2}$ (this is not entirely correct according to the section in the text on the effective concentration in vivo*). After 24 h (i.e. six times the elimination half-life of HBOP to the left) REIT declined only to about 30%. After 2 days ($12 \times t_{1/2}$) there are still 10% REIT left.*

(where IC_{50} = concentration of the β-adrenoceptor blocking drug which causes half-maximal effect). The linearization is only valid within the bonds $0 \cdot 2 \times E_{max} <$ REHR, REIT $< 0 \cdot 8 \times E_{max}$ (Fig. 1). Moreover, the E_{max} model itself is just another formulation of the general 'law of mass action' which also governs the receptor binding kinetics. In this context, Wellstein and colleagues (9) recently supported the validity of the E_{max} model (and its linearization) for the *in vivo* effects of β-adrenoceptor blocking drugs. They demonstrated that the receptor occupancy in an *in vitro* RRA of active drug in plasma samples, predicted accurately the reduction in heart rate at the time the plasma sample was drawn. In healthy subjects taking propranolol the prediction was best in the case of orthostasis-induced heart rate where the sensitivity parameter of the RRA, K_i, was equal to the *in vivo* IC_{50} value.

Explanation of the long-lasting reduction in heart rate

Clinical data

The equations discussed above make it clear that REHR and REIT decrease slower than the plasma concentration and that this is true for all β-adrenoceptor blockers.

However, in the case of BOP, these effects decline exceptionally slowly. After an oral dose of 4 mg BOP significant effects (REHR) compared to placebo were measured in healthy subjects up to 96 h (1). After giving 2 mg doses until steady state was reached, the peak effect, 50% REIT, was reached 3 h after the last dose. Sixty-nine hours later, there were still 8% REIT left (3). Even 24 h after a single oral dose of 1 mg an effect of 8·2% REHR was measurable. This compares to a peak effect of 20% REHR at 3 h (2).

High potency and shallow slope

Several clinical trials compared BOP with other β-adrenoceptor antagonists. Schiess and co-workers (10) showed at several dose levels, that y mg BOP were as potent as $7{\cdot}5 \times y$ mg pindolol and $50 \times y$ mg atenolol in the treatment of essential hypertension. In the same indication BOP was as potent as 100 times the dose of metoprolol (11). These findings support the statement about the high potency of BOP ($K_D = 0{\cdot}1$ nmol/1) made earlier.

The flatter the concentration-effect (REHR, REIT) curve, i.e. the smaller its slope, the longer the effect will persist while plasma concentrations are decreasing. This principle is illustrated in Fig. 1 for BOP. A comparison with other β-adrenoceptor antagonists shows that BOP displays the shallowest slope (12). It is interesting to note that BOP also possesses intrinsic sympathomimetic activity, ISA, (13) and investigators have speculated about a causal relationship with the flat slope of the REHR, REIT-concentration curve (13,14).

Besides prolonging the action a shallow slope generates a buffer between pharmacokinetic and pharmacodynamic variability. It is therefore not surprising that in a study of BOP, with extensive and poor metabolizers of the dibrisoquine-sparteine type significant differences were only found in the concentration-time profiles but not in the effect (REIT)-time profiles (15). This buffer obviously also alleviates the consequences of occasional non-compliance with the dosing regimen.

Figure 1 shows graphically how high potency and a shallow slope collaborate to generate the long-lasting effect in REIT after a single oral dose of 2 mg BOP, which generates a C_{max} well above the IC_{50}. Even when 12 elimination half-lives (12×4 h) have passed, after C_{max} had been reached, 10% of the REIT still remains.

By connecting the pharmacokinetic with the pharmacodynamic model Platzer and colleagues (3) could accurately predict the steady state effect-time profile of 2 mg BOP once daily using parameters estimated from single dose data. This proves that:

1. the pharmacokinetic model is adequate (no deep compartment with $t_{1/2} > 4$ h);
2. the effect (REIT) does not accumulate, a finding which rules out irreversible receptor binding of HBOP;
3. there are no other active metabolites, besides HBOP, with longer elimination half-lives. Therefore, the simple relationship presented in Fig. 1 is also valid to predict effects from steady state concentrations.

Conclusions

The long duration of reduction of stimulated heart rate in healthy subjects is a consequence of the high potency of BOP and the shallow slope of the concentration-effect relationship. An elimination half-life of 4 h of HBOP from plasma ensures that there is no accumulation of drug after repeated once daily doses. A remarkably large therapeutic index allows dosing for several days at once. Doses as high as 12 mg were tolerated well by healthy subjects (1). Dosage of 8 mg once weekly was as effective and safe as 1 mg once daily in the treatment of hypertension (11). The shallow slope of the concentration-effect relationship acts as a buffer between pharmacokinetics and -dynamics and alleviates the consequences of occasional non-compliance with the dosing regimen. Apart from the possibility of dosing BOP according to the patient's preference (once daily, every second day or even once a week) there seems to be no basic therapeutic advantage from the long duration of action in the treatment of hypertension (10).

References

(1) Aellig WH. Pharmacological experiments in healthy volunteers with bopindolol, a long-acting beta-adrenoceptor blocking drug with partial agonist activity. *Br J Clin Pharmacol* 1985; **19**: 775–781.

(2) Aellig WH, Nüesch E, Engel G, Grevel J, Niederberger W, Rosenthaler J. Relationship between plasma levels and cardiac beta-adrenoceptor blockade: a study with oral and intravenous bopindolol. *Br J Clin Pharmacol* 1986; **21**: 45–51.

(3) Platzer R, Galeazzi RL, Niederberger W, Rosenthaler J. Simultaneous modelling of bopindolol kinetics and dynamics. *Clin Pharmacol Ther* 1984; **36**: 5–13.

(4) Johnsson G, Regårdh CG. Clinical pharmacokinetics of beta-adrenoceptor blocking drugs. *Clin Pharmacokin* 1876; **1**: 253–263.

(5) Kumana CR, Kaye CM. An investigation of the relationship between beta-adrenoceptor blockade and plasma practolol concentration in man. *Eur J Clin Pharmacol* 1984; **7**: 243–248.

(6) Maronde RF, Robinson D, Vlachakis ND *et al.* Study of single and multiple dose pharmacokinetic/pharmacodynamic modelling of the antihypertensive effects of labetalol. *Am J Med* 1983; **75**: 40–47.

(7) Campbell DB, Drew M, Chignon JC. Prediction of the prolonged *in vivo* beta-blockade by tertatolol from plasma concentrations and *in vitro* receptor binding studies. *Br J Clin Pharmacol* 1986; **22**: 205P.

(8) Coltart DJ, Shand DG. Plasma propranolol levels in the quantitative assessment of beta-adrenergic blockade in man. *Br Med J* 1970; **3**: 731–734.

(9) Wellstein A, Palm D, Pitschner HF, Belz GC. Receptor binding of propranolol is the missing link between plasma concentration kinetics and the effect-time course in man. *Eur J Clin Pharmacol* 1985; **29**: 131–147.

(10) Schiess W, Welzel D, Gugler R. Double-blind comparison of once-daily bopindolol, pindolol and atenolol in essential hypertension. *Eur J Clin Pharmacol* 1984; **27**: 529–534.

(11) Andersson OK, Hedner T, Nyberg G. Acute and long-term antihypertensive effect of bopindolol—a nonselective beta-adrenergic blocker with ISA. *Eur J Clin Pharmacol* 1985; **29**: 281–285.

(12) Grevel J. Pharmacodynamic models of various beta-blockers: An explanation for the long duration of action of bopindolol. *J Cardiovasc Pharmacol* 1986; (in press).

(13) Nyberg G. Intrinsic sympathomimetic activity of bopindolol, a non-selective beta-adrenoceptor antagonist. *Br J Clin Pharmacol* 1985; **20**: 242.

(14) Carruthers SG, Pacha WL, Aellig WH. Contrasts between pindolol and propranolol concentration-response relationships. *Br J Clin Pharmacol* 1985; **20**: 417–420.

(15) Dayer P, Marmy A, Leemann T, Rosenthaler J, Fabre J. Interindividual variability in beta-adrenoceptor blocking drug behaviour—a comparison of atenolol, bopindolol and metoprolol. *Kidney Int* 1984; **24**: 984.

Antihypertensive and metabolic effects of bopindolol at rest and during exercise — is once weekly dosage possible?

O. K. ANDERSSON,[1] T. HEDNER[2] and G. NYBERG[3]

[1]*Department of Medicine I, Sahlgrenska Hospital, Göteborg*
[2]*Department ofClinical Pharmacology, Sahlgrenska Hospital, Göteborg*
[3]*Department of Medicine, Östra Hospital, Göteborg, Sweden*

Summary

Fourteen male hypertensive patients, mean age 53 years, first took part in a 3-month, double-blind crossover comparison of 1–2 mg bopindolol, a non-selective β-blocker with ISA, and 100–200 mg metoprolol. Effects on blood pressure and heart rate as well as electrolytes, blood glucose, lactate, free fatty acids and circulating noradrenaline were followed at rest and during standardized exercise. One patient dropped out after the initial phase and the remaining 13 patients were followed for 1 year on bopindolol. Eight hypertensives measured blood pressure at home, and in these patients bopindololl mg once daily and 8 mg once weekly were compared in a double-blind fashion, for 3 weeks on each regimen.

Bopindolol in a mean dose of 1·35 mg/day caused a significant reduction in blood pressure (26/15 mmHg), as did metoprolol (24/13 mmHg) in a mean dose of 144 mg/day. These doses caused similar inhibition of exercise tachycardia. During submaximal exercise, similar and expected effects on lactate and FFA were noted, but glucose concentrations were significantly reduced on bopindolol. The increase in S-potassium during exercise was normalized within 5 min rest on both drugs and circulating noradrenaline was equally increased during exercise on both drugs and placebo. During long-term therapy with bopindolol, satisfactory blood pressure control was maintained for up to 1 year in all patients, the average supine blood pressure being reduced from 173/107 to 144/90 mmHg. During treatment with 8 mg bopindolol once weekly blood pressure control was satisfactorily maintained during the week and no significant difference was observed in comparison with daily administration (1 mg) of the drug.

Thus, effective blood pressure control was achieved with bopindolol in patients with mild hypertension. The effect was sustained over 12 months and tolerance was

The position of bopindolol, a new β-blocker, edited by P. A. van Zwieten, 1987: Royal Society of Medicine Services International Congress and Symposium Series No. 106, published by Royal Society of Medicine Services Limited.

good. The relatively long half-life of the drug made it possible to use it in a once weekly regimen.

Introduction

Bopindolol (LT 31-200: 4-(2-benzoyloxy-3-tert-butylaminopropoxy)-2-methyl indate: Sandoz AG, Basle Switzerland) is a new, long-acting, non-selective, β-adrenoceptor antagonist. Animal pharmacological studies have indicated a mild membrane stabilizing effect and moderate intrinsic sympathomimetic activity (ISA) (3). In one particular study of healthy volunteers, however, the ISA was shown to be approximately of the same magnitude as that of pindolol (7). High potency and long duration of action of bopindolol on inhibition of exercise tachycardia had been reported earlier (1,9). From these studies it was anticipated that at the peak effect 1 mg bopindolol would cause a similar reduction of exercise tachycardia as that of 100 mg metoprolol. In an open study, bopindolol 1–4 mg given once daily to hypertensive patients effectively reduced blood pressure and heart rate over a 12-week treatment period (4).

The purpose of the present study was to investigate in patients with mild to moderate hypertension whether a) bopindolol and metoprolol, in doses equipotent with regard to inhibition of exercise tachycardia, would produce a similar antihypertensive effect, b) long-term bopindolol treatment for 1 year was effective and well tolerated, and c) satisfactory blood pressure control could be maintained by giving the total 7-day dose only once a week, d) any metabolic differences could be detected between metoprolol and bopindolol, at rest or during exercise.

Patients and methods

Patients

Fourteen male patients with essential hypertension who had not been treated previously were selected for the initial crossover part of the study. Secondary forms of hypertension were excluded (2). Inclusion blood pressures (BP) were: diastolic (DBP) $\geq 95 \leq 125$ mmHg and systolic (SBP) such that mean arterial (MAP) was ≥ 117 mmHg for those aged 30–39, and ≥ 127 mmHg for those of 40–59 years; the mean age was 54 years (range 35–63 years) and ten patients were classified as WHO Stage 1 and four as WHO Stage 2. Mean weight was 86·7 kg (range 67·1–114·0 kg). Informed consent was given by the patients before inclusion and approval was obtained from the Ethics Committee of the University of Göteborg.

Methods

The first part of the study (Fig. 1) was designed as a double-blind, crossover comparison of bopindolol (dose range 1–2 mg daily) and metoprolol (dose range 100–200 mg daily) followed by an open evaluation of bopindolol for 1 year ($n = 13$). At the end of the 1-year evaluation, the patients were trained to measure blood pressure

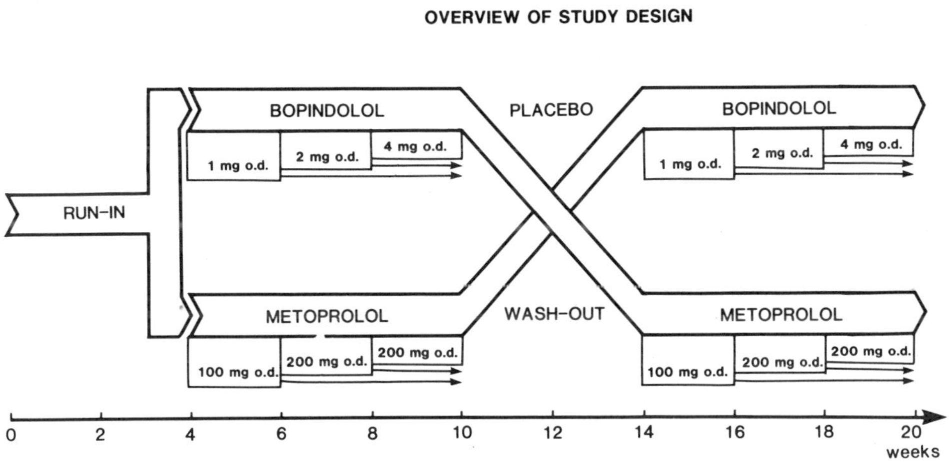

Figure 1. Design of the study.

at home and eight patients learned the method satisfactorily. They were included in a 6-week double-blind comparison of bopindolol 1 mg once daily and 8 mg once weekly. At the end of each treatment period during the initial acute crossover trial a bicycle ergometer test (Elema-Schonander electrically braked bicycle, Eo22E) was performed. The exercise was started at 50 Watt for 2 min, then the load was increased by 10 Watt every 2 min to a final work load of 100 Watt. The total exercise time was 30 min: blood pressure and heart rate (BP and HR) were measured at each step.

Blood samples for special biochemical tests (noradrenaline, glucose, free fatty acid and lactate) were drawn after 30 min supine rest before the ergometer test, after 15 and 30 min of dynamic exercise and at 5, 15 and 30 min of supine rest after the exercise test. Plasma catecholamines were analyzed with an HPLC method with electrochemical capture (6) and glucose, lactate and FFA according to automatic routine procedures.

In the initial double-blind evaluation, BP and HR were measured blindly with a semiautomatic manometer (Auto-Manometer, 8). During the rest of the study BP and HR were measured at 11 h 00–12 h 00 by a research nurse using a standard mercury sphygmomanometer. At home, BP and HR were measured with the patient sitting, in the morning immediately before tablet intake. The measurements were performed by auscultation with an anaeroid sphygmomanometer. All BP evaluations took Korotkoff Phase I as SBP and Phase V as DBP.

In the crossover and long-term evaluation studies the trial preparations were given in the morning as capsules containing either placebo, 1 mg bopindolol or 100 mg metoprolol. The doses were increased after 2 weeks if target pressures were not reached (DBP $\leq$ 90 mmHg and MAP $\leq$ 110 mmHg for the age group 30–39 years, and DBP $\leq$ 95 mmHg and MAP $\leq$ 117 mmHg for the age group 40–65 years. The maximum doses were 2 mg bopindolol and 200 mg metoprolol. During the once daily vs once weekly double-blind comparison, capsules were given each morning for periods of 3 weeks. The capsules contained either 1 mg bopindolol, which was taken regularly, or 8 mg bopindolol, which was administered at the start of the week followed by placebo capsules each day.

The statistical significance of differences from values obtained with placebo treatment were calculated by analysis of variance with two independent criteria for classification, followed by Student's *t*-test (5). Differences were regarded as significant when $p < 0{\cdot}05$.

Results

Bopindolol vs metoprolol

During the run-in period the patients showed a stable blood pressure level in the supine position (Fig. 1). Immediately prior to the crossover study the mean supine SBP was 173 ± 3 mmHg (m ± SEM). DBP was 106 ± 1 mmHg, and the heart rate was 79 ± 4 beats/min. During the wash-out period supine SBP and DBP amounted to 169 ± 4 and 102 ± 1 mmHg, respectively and HR: 76 ± 2 beats/min. In comparison with the run-in period, there was a significant reduction in supine BP during bopindolol treatment: SBP was 143 ± 4 ($p<0{\cdot}001$), DPB was 87 ± 2 mmHg ($p<0{\cdot}001$) and HR was 61 ± beats/min ($p<0{\cdot}001$). During metoprolol treatment significant reductions were observed in supine BP. SBP was 145 ± 5 ($p<0{\cdot}001$) DBP was 89 ± 3 mmHg ($p<0{\cdot}001$) and HR was 64 ± 3 beats/min ($p<0{\cdot}001$). Hence the reduction in BP was comparable for both drugs and so was the reduction in HR. In the standing position similar and significant reductions in SBP, DBP and HR were seen after bopindolol and metoprolol. No orthostatic hypotensive reaction was observed.

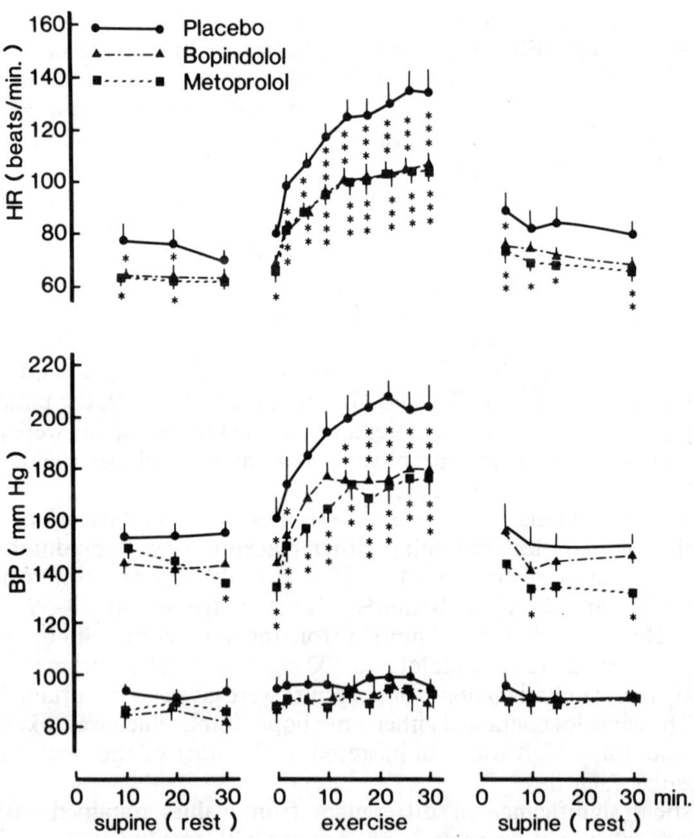

Figure 2. Heart rate (HR) and systolic blood pressure (BP) during supine rest and bicycle ergometry on placebo, bopindolol and metoprolol.

Submaximal exercise test

The results of BP and HR from the bicycle ergometry tests are given in Fig. 2: HR as well as SBP were significantly reduced during treatment with both bopindolol and metoprolol, compared to double-blind placebo values. The reduction of exercise-induced tachycardia was similar at both treatment schedules and at 30 min exercise HR was reduced by 36 ± 4 beats/min with bopindolol and by 35 ± 6 beats/min with metoprolol (NS).

Metabolic evaluation during exercise

Biochemical tests performed before, during and after dynamic exercise included plasma potassium (Table 1), glucose (Table 2), lactate (Table 3), free fatty acids (Table 4) and noradrenaline (Table 5).

The apparent changes during exercise in potassium lactate, free fatty acids and noradrenaline were similar for all treatments and did not differ significantly. Plasma glucose changes were more pronounced with bopindolol. The decrease during exercise was significant with bopindolol but not with placebo or metoprolol.

Table 1

Metabolic effects of bopindolol or metoprolol during exercise and rest

Plasma potassium (mmol/l)	Placebo	Metoprolol	Bopindolol
Resting supine	3·85 ± 0·15	4·09 ± 0·26	3·90 ± 0·22
Bicycle ergometry			
(min) 15	4·43 ± 0·32	4·46 ± 0·24	4·61 ± 0·28
30	4·52 ± 0·22	4·77 ± 0·29	4·79 ± 0·28
Postexercise rest			
(min) 5	4·11 ± 0·18	4·29 ± 0·29	4·29 ± 0·16
15	4·11 ± 0·12	4·11 ± 0·25	4·16 ± 0·20
30	3·94 ± 0·21	4·13 ± 0·24	4·20 ± 0·33

Shown are means ± SEM $n = 8$

Table 2

Metabolic effects of bopindolol or metoprolol during exercise and rest

Blood glucose (mmol/l)	Placebo	Metoprolol	Bopindolol
Resting supine	4·58 ± 0·38	4·33 ± 0·40	4·88 ± 0·38
Bicycle ergometry			
(min) 15	4·23 ± 0·52	4·49 ± 0·43	4·33 ± 0·45*
30	4·26 ± 0·54	4·15 ± 0·40	4·00 ± 0·74**
Postexercise rest			
(min) 5	4·23 ± 0·65	4·36 ± 0·44	4·34 ± 0·73
15	4·34 ± 0·49	4·36 ± 0·41	4·23 ± 0·69
30	4·26 ± 0·71	4·61 ± 1·40	4·27 ± 0·57

Shown are means ± SEM $n = 8$
*$p < 0.05$
**$p < 0.01$

Table 3

Metabolic effects of bopindolol or metoprolol during exercise and rest

Blood lactate (mmol/l)	Placebo	Metoprolol	Bopindolol
Resting supine	0·99±0·31	0·88±0·32	0·93±0·21
Bicycle ergometry			
(min) 15	2·09±1·48	2·08±1·19	2·08±0·79
30	2·61±2·04	2·49±1·71	2·33±1·37
Postexercise rest			
(min) 5	2·13±1·44	2·06±1·38	2·16±1·38
15	1·33±0·70	1·50±0·95	1·54±0·94
30	1·40±1·10	1·12±0·58	1·49±1·46

Shown are means ± SEM $n=8$

Table 4

Metabolic effects of bopindolol or metoprolol during exercise and rest

Plasma fatty acid (mmol/l)	Placebo	Metoprolol	Bopindolol
Resting supine	0·56±0·41	1·01±0·75	0·58±0·27
Bicycle ergometry			
(min) 15	0·64±0·46	0·93±0·81	0·43±0·26
30	1·08±0·73	1·17±0·80	0·89±0·34
Postexercise rest			
(min) 5	1·36±0·62	1·36±0·74	1·15±0·43
15	1·41±0·60	1·59±0·63	1·18±0·44
30	1·13±0·69	1·30±0·79	0·93±0·37

Shown are means ± SEM $n=8$

Table 5

Metabolic effects of bopindolol or metoprolol during exercise and rest

Noradrenaline (mg/ml)	Placebo	Metoprolol	Bopindolol
Resting supine	0·40±0·05	0·43±0·06	0·28±0·07
Bicycle ergometry			
(min) 30	1·01±0·14	1·21±0·13	1·21±0·30
Postexercise rest			
(min) 15	0·47±0·05	0·47±0·04	0·35±0·09
30	0·41±0·06	0·43±0·04	0·32±0·09

Shown are means ± SEM $n=8$

Long-term bopindolol therapy

The BP reduction in the open long-term study was evaluated every third month and compared with the run-in BP (173 ± 3/107 ± 1 mmHg). A highly significant reduction in BP was observed during the first 3–6 months, when the supine BP level was reasonably constant, namely 154 ± 5/93 ± 2 mmHg and 153 ± 5/95 ± 2 mmHg, respectively. A minor drop in BP was also observed between the sixth month

(153 ± 3/95 ± 3 mmHg) and the ninth month (143 ± 3/91 ± 2 mmHg) in spite of the unchanged dose of bopindolol and HR fell significantly from 79·3 ± 4·1 (control) to 69 ± 3 beats/min 12 months after initiation of therapy.

Bopindolol once daily vs once weekly

When comparing sitting BP and HR measured at home on different dose regimens, it was apparent that during therapy with bopindolol 8 mg once weekly the BP level was well maintained in comparison with the result on 1 mg daily. The BP at the end of each of 3 treatment weeks was 146 ± 5/97 ± 4, 141 ± 6/90 ± 5 and 143 ± 7/96 ± 5 mmHg when bopindolol was taken as an 8 mg dose at the start of each week. The corresponding BPs were 139 ± 5/97 ± 4, 142 ± 6/95 ± 5 and 143 ± 4/92 ± 4 mmHg when bopindolol was administered 1 mg daily. No significant difference in HR was observed. 2·4 and 8 weeks after cessation of the therapy BP was 151 ± 3/96 ± 2, 158 ± 3/98 ± 2 and 165 ± 2/104 ± 1 mmHg, respectively. HR has regained pretreatment values 2 weeks after withdrawal.

Discussion

In the initial crossover study with treatment periods of 6 weeks mean SBP and DBP did not differ between bopindolol (mean dose 1·35 mg/day) and metoprolol (mean dose 144 mg/day) treatments either in the supine or standing positions. These doses were chosen as inhibition of exercise tachycardia was expected and found to be identical for the two drugs (Fig. 2). Thus, with comparable β-adrenergic blockade at a dose ratio of approximately 1 : 100, the two drugs were equipotent with respect to blood pressure control at rest.

The results of the comparison of once daily and once weekly dosing are interesting, since they showed that a single weekly dose which was well tolerated and which did not cause an undue reduction in heart rate and blood pressure during its peak effect, was able to maintain blood pressure control. It may be argued, that the self-measured blood pressures were not comparable to the readings made in the clinic, and that the latter measurements may induce a higher 'stress' level in the subjects. However, when the two sets of values were compared, the average values did not differ from what was found at the end of treatment for 1 year. Sitting diastolic blood pressure at home averaged 3–4 mmHg higher than the pressures in the clinic. In the standing position the reverse was seen.

Although once weekly administration of antihypertensive therapy is not presently proposed as therapy, its adoption might well improve compliance in certain patients even over once daily treatment. A large weekly dose of a long-acting drug may cause long-lasting adverse effects, but this possibility could largely be eliminated by first establishing that tolerance is good with once daily therapy, and then gradually increasing the dose and changing to once weekly dosing in selected cases. On the other hand, if adverse effects occur, an agent with a long duration of action would be less desirable than a more short-acting substance.

References

(1) Aellig WH. Pharmacological experiments in healthy volunteers with bopindolol, a long-acting β-adrenoceptor blocking drug with partial agonist activity. *Br J Clin Pharmacol* 1985; **19**: 775–781.

(2) Andersson OK, Berglund G, Hansson L, Sannerstedt R, Sivertsson R, Wikstrand J, Wilhelmsson L. Organization and efficacy of an outpatient hypertension clinic. *Acta Med Scand* 1978; **203**: 391–398.

(3) Berthold R, Waite R, Weber H. Pharmacological studies with bopindolol: a new long acting β-adrenoceptor antagonist. *Br J Pharmacol* 1981; **74**: 829.

(4) van Brummelen P, Bühler FR, Amann FW, Bolli P. Effects of a new long-acting beta-blocker bopindolol (LT 31-200) on blood pressure, plasma catecholamines, renin and cholesterol in patients with arterial hypertension. *Eur J Clin Pharmacol* 1982; **22**: 491–493.

(5) Davies OL. (1949). Statistical methods in research and production. London: Oliver and Boyd.

(6) Hjemdal P, Daleskog M, Kahan T. Determination of plasma catecholamines by high performance liquid chromatography with electrochemical detection: comparison with a radioenzymatic method. *Life Sci* 1979; **25**, 131–138.

(7) Nyberg G. Intrinsic sympathomimetic activity of bopindolol, a nonselective β-adrenergic antagonist. *Br J Clin Pharmacol* 1985; (in press).

(8) Nyberg G. Indirect blood pressure and heart rate measured quickly without observer bias using a semiautomatic machine (Auto-Manometer)—response to isometric exercise in normally healthy males and its modification by β-adrenoceptor blockage. *Br J Clin Pharmacol* 1979; **4**: 275–281.

(9) Turner DR, Goodwin FJ, Knight AR, Littlejohns DW, Sharman VI. Vere DW. Bopindolol: A new long acting β-receptor antagonist: its effects on hemodynamics, and on the renin response to tilting. *Br J Clin Pharmacol* 1984; **17**: 295–299.

Bopindolol induced changes in plasma lipid fractions in hypertensive patients

P. VAN BRUMMELEN[1] **and F. R. BÜHLER**[2]

Department of Nephrology, University Hospital, Leiden, The Netherlands[1]
Department of Medicine, University Hospital, Basel, Switzerland[2]

Summary

The influence of monotherapy with the new betablocker bopindolol on the plasma levels of total cholesterol, triglycerides, low density lipoprotein cholesterol and high density lipoprotein cholesterol was investigated in 24 patients with mild to moderate essential hypertension. Bopindolol 1–4 mg daily lowered blood pressure and heart rate significantly. In 18 of 24 patients diastolic blood pressure was lowered to values <95 mmHg. When compared with placebo no changes were found in the plasma levels of total cholesterol, low density lipoprotein cholesterol and high density lipoprotein cholesterol after 4, 8 and 12 weeks of treatment with bopindolol. Plasma triglycerides increased significantly after 4 and 8 weeks of treatment but after 12 weeks of treatment the difference with placebo was no longer significant. Side effects were minimal and in no instance did treatment have to be discontinued. It is concluded that bopindolol is an effective and well tolerated β-blocker in hypertensive patients. The finding that it does not lower high density lipoprotein cholesterol could be a potential advantage.

Introduction

The finding that several antihypertensive drugs, apart from lowering blood pressure, also influence plasma lipid concentrations has recently received ample attention (1,2). For diuretics and most β-blockers, the change in plasma lipids is in an unfavourable direction, and it has been suggested that this could potentially limit the benefit derived from their antihypertensive action (2). Especially the relative lack of effectiveness of antihypertensive treatment in preventing ischaemic heart disease has been putatively attributed to this metabolic side-effect (2,3). In one of the first clinical trials on the effectiveness and tolerability of the β-blocker bopindolol a statistical significant

The position of bopindolol, a new β-blocker, edited by P. A. van Zwieten, 1987: Royal Society of Medicine Services International Congress and Symposium Series No. 106, published by Royal Society of Medicine Services Limited.

reduction in plasma cholesterol was found (4). It was felt, however, that further studies on greater numbers of patients and including the measurement of lipoprotein fractions were needed to confirm or deny this possible favourable action of bopindolol with regard to plasma lipids. Here we report on the effects of this new long acting β-adrenoceptor blocker with partial agonist activity on plasma lipids in hypertensive patients.

Patients and methods

Twenty-four patients with mild to moderate essential hypertension (19 males and 5 females, aged 20–60 years) were investigated. In the patients who had been treated previously all medication was withdrawn. All patients gave informed consent.

After a placebo period of 4–6 weeks, active treatment with bopindolol 1 mg once daily was started. When necessary this dosage was increased at bi-weekly intervals to 2 or 4 mg bopindolol once daily until a diastolic blood pressure of 95 mmHg was achieved. When, after 4 weeks on 4 mg bopindolol the diastolic blood pressure was >95 mmHg, the patient was withdrawn from the study. In the other patients the minimal effective dose of bopindolol was given for a total period of 12 weeks.

Blood pressure and heart rate in the sitting position and body weight were measured at all visits. Blood for determination of plasma lipids and lipoprotein fractions was drawn from the fasting patient at the end of the placebo period and after 4, 8 and 12 weeks on the final dose of bopindolol. Total cholesterol and triglyceride concentrations were estimated with the fully automatical enzymatic SMAC method. Very low density lipoproteins (VLDL) were separated by preparative ultracentrifugation and VLDL cholesterol and triglyceride concentrations were estimated with enzymatic methods. High density lipoprotein (HDL) cholesterol concentration was measured by precipitation of VLDL and LDL with $MnCl_2$ and heparin and subsequent measurement of cholesterol in the supernatant fluid (5), LDL cholesterol concentrations were then calculated by subtracting VLDL cholesterol and HDL cholesterol from total cholesterol. The results are presented as mean values ± standard deviation (SD). For evaluations of statistical significance the paired *t*-test was used.

Results

Bopindolol reduced the systolic and diastolic blood pressure significantly (Table 1). In 18 patients a diastolic blood pressure <95 mmHg was achieved, in four patients when on 1 mg, in five patients when on 2 mg and in nine patients when on 4 mg bopindolol. In six of the 24 patients the goal blood pressure was not reached. Heart rate was reduced by bopindolol. Changes in body weight were small (Table 1). Bopindolol treatment was well tolerated. Side-effects volunteered were vivid dreams (two cases), cold extremities (one case), muscle cramps (one case) and diarrhoea (one case). All were slight and in no instance did treatment have to be discontinued.

Plasma concentrations of total cholesterol, LDL cholesterol and HDL cholesterol remained unchanged during treatment with bopindolol (Table 2). The plasma concentration of triglycerides was increased by 41% after 4 weeks on the final dose of bopindolol. Hereafter it appeared to decrease and after 12 weeks the difference with the placebo value (+24%) was no longer statistically significant (Table 2).

Table 1

Sitting systolic and diastolic blood pressure, heart rate and body weight during placebo and during bopindolol treatment

	Placebo	Bopindolol		
		4	8	12 weeks
	($n=24$)	($n=24$)	($n=18$)	($n=12$)
Systolic blood pressure (mmHg)	158 ± 16	141 ± 19**	139 ± 10**	135 ± 11**
Diastolic blood pressure (mmHg)	105 ± 7	94 ± 11**	91 ± 6**	86 ± 6**
Pulse rate beats/min)	74 ± 11	66 ± 9*	65 ± 10*	65 ± 10*
Body weight (kg)	75 ± 26	76 ± 17	80 ± 14	80 ± 14

Data are given as mean values ± SD. Statistical significance of differences with placebo treatment *$p<0{\cdot}01$, **$p<0{\cdot}001$.

Table 2

Plasma lipid fractions during placebo and during bopindolol treatment

	Placebo	Bopindolol		
		4	8	12 weeks
	($n=24$)	($n=24$)	($n=18$)	($n=18$)
Total cholesterol (mmol/l)	5·39 ± 0·25	5·37 ± 0·22	5·55 ± 0·31	5·33 ± 0·33
LDL cholesterol (mmol/l)	3·65 ± 1·14	3·39 ± 0·94	3·64 ± 1·06	3·39 ± 1·00
HDL cholesterol (mmol/l)	1·33 ± 0·30	1·33 ± 0·41	1·27 ± 0·29	1·30 ± 0·41
Triglycerides	1·35 ± 0·19	1·90 ± 0·25**	1·84 ± 0·26	1·68 ± 0·31

Data are given as mean values ± SD. Statistical significance of differences with placebo treatment *$p<0{\cdot}02$, **$p<0{\cdot}01$.

Discussion

The antihypertensive efficacy and good tolerance of bopindolol as reported by us in two earlier studies (4,6) was confirmed in the present investigation. In addition, it was found that bopindolol did not influence the plasma concentrations of total cholesterol or its main fraction, LDL cholesterol. Our earlier finding of a decrease in total cholesterol concentration during bopindolol treatment (4) could not be verified in this study which included a greater number of patients. With the exception of sotalol, β-blockers do not influence total cholesterol or LDL cholesterol (7,8). In most studies on the influence of β-blocker therapy on plasma lipids increases in triglycerides have been found and here the same is shown for bopindolol. The increase was statistically significant after 4 and 8 weeks but smaller and not-significant after 12 weeks of treatment. It would require a study of still longer duration to determine whether the effect on plasma triglycerides tapers off gradually or, alternatively, that the observed differences are due to physiological fluctuations. In favour of the first view would be the observation of Berglund and Andersson (9) that after 6 years of propranolol treatment in hypertensive patients plasma triglycerides were only slightly and non-significantly above pretreatment level. Apart from the duration of treatment also the type of β-blocker seems to be of relevance (8). Most β-blockers have been reported to lower HDL cholesterol (7,8) but in the present study the plasma concentration of HDL cholesterol was not changed by bopindolol treatment.

With regard to the underlying mechanisms, it has recently been suggested that the β-blocker-induced changes in both triglycerides and HDL cholesterol are the result of inhibition of lipoprotein lipase by predominantly α-adrenergic stimulation (10), but other explanations have not been excluded.

Long-term, large-scale clinical trials are necessary to establish the clinical significance of drug-induced changes in plasma lipids. In our opinion it seems prudent, as long as the innocent nature of these changes has not been established, to extrapolate from epidemiological data and to consider this aspect when choosing between the various antihypertensive drugs. Bopindolol may offer some potential advantage in this respect by not lowering HDL cholesterol.

References

(1) Johnson BF. The emerging problem of plasma lipid changes during antihypertensive therapy. *J Cardiovasc Pharmacol* 1982; **4**(suppl): S213–221.

(2) Anonymous. Antihypertensive drugs, plasma lipids, and coronary disease (Editorial). *Lancet* 1980; **ii**: 19–20.

(3) Leren P, Foss PO, Helgeland A, Hjermann I, Holme I, Lund-Larsen PG. Effect of propranolol and prazosin on blood lipids. The Oslo Study. *Lancet* 1980; **ii**: 4–6.

(4) Van Brummelen P, Bühler FR, Amann FW, Bolli P. Effects of a new long-acting betablocker bopindolol (LT 31–200) on blood pressure, plasma catecholamines, renin and cholesterol in patients with arterial hypertension. *Eur J Clin Pharmacol* 1982; **22**: 491–493.

(5) Burstein M, Scholnick HR, Morfin R. Rapid method for the isolation of lipoproteins from human serum by precipitation with polyanions. *J Lipid Res* 1970; **11**: 583.

(6) Hulthen UL, Van Brummelen P, Amann FW, Bühler FR. Antihypertensive efficacy of the new long acting betablocker bopindolol as related to age. *J Cardiovasc Pharmacol* 1983; **5**: 426–429.

(7) Johnson BF. The emerging problem of plasma lipid changes during antihypertensive therapy. *J Cardiovasc Pharmacol* 1982; **4**(suppl 2): S213–S221.

(8) Van Brummelen P. The relevance of intrinsic sympathomimetic activity for betablocker-induced changes in plasma lipids. *J Cardiovasc Pharmacol* 1983; **5**: S51–S55.

(9) Berglund G, Andersson O. Beta-blockers or diuretics in hypertension? A six year follow-up of blood pressure and metabolic side effects. *Lancet* 1981; **i**: 744–747.

(10) Day JL, Metcalfe J, Simpson CN. Adrenergic mechanisms in control of plasma lipid concentrations. *Br Med J* 1982; **284**: 1145–1148.

Age-independence of the antihypertensive efficacy of β-blocker treatment

PETER WEIDMANN, JEAN-CHARLES BOUSQUET and THE SWISS PRACTITIONERS BOPINDOLOL STUDY GROUP

Medizinische Poliklinik, Universität von Bern, die Schweiz

Summary

β-Blockers are now well established as alternative first line drugs for treating hypertension. Bopindolol is a new β-blocker with a long duration of action and antihypertensive properties at low dosage. To assess the blood pressure (BP)-lowering effect and tolerance of bopindolol, 655 hypertensive patients with diastolic BP > 100 mmHg (age 22–80 years; mean ± SD, 51 ± 10 years) were evaluated prospectively by a study group of practising physicians. Following discontinuation of previous antihypertensive drugs for 4 weeks and/or a 2-week placebo phase, bopindolol, 1 mg/day, was given for 12 weeks. Bopindolol dose was decreased to 0·5 mg/day if diastolic BP after 8 weeks was ≤ 85 mmHg; chlorthalidone, 12·5–25 mg/day, was added if diastolic BP was ≥ 95 mmHg after 4 or 8 weeks of bopindolol monotherapy.

Compared to placebo, BP was lowered ($p < 0·0001$) by bopindolol monotherapy (patients, $n = 302$) from 160/104 ± 14/4 to 139/89 ± 13·6 mmHg, by combination treatment (patients, $n = 320$) from 166/108 ± 16/6 to 145/95 ± 15/7 mmHg. Diastolic BP was reduced to < 95 mmHg by bopindolol 0·5 or 1 mg/day in 265 patients, by combination treatment in 167 patients. Bopindolol-induced absolute or percentage decreases in systolic or diastolic BP did not correlate with age ($r = -0·07$–$0·10$). Heart rate was decreased ($p < 0·0001$) from 77 ± 10 to 68 ± 8 beats/min. Subjective side effects on active treatment occurred after 4 weeks in 18·2%, after 12 weeks in 15·1%. However, such symptoms led to interruption of treatment in 4·9% of patients only, and the total incidence and the severity of complaints were largely unchanged or even decreased during active treatment as compared to placebo. Body weight and serum creatinine were largely unchanged; while serum uric acid was increased slightly on combination treatment and minimally on bopindolol monotherapy. Serum potassium was decreased minimally on combination therapy (4·37–4·00 mmol/l).

These findings demonstrate that bopindolol is a useful agent for the treatment of various age groups with hypertension in general practice.

The position of bopindolol, a new β-blocker, edited by P. A. van Zwieten, 1987: Royal Society of Medicine Services International Congress and Symposium Series No. 106, published by Royal Society of Medicine Services Limited.

Introduction

β-blockers are well established as useful alternative agents for the first line treatment of essential hypertension. Compared with the more conventional diuretic therapy, the antihypertensive potency and subjective tolerance of various β-blockers seem to be on average quite similar (1–4). Nevertheless, additional characteristics may influence the practical choice among such drugs. Diuretics exert more metabolic side-effects than β-blockers (1,4–8). There are suggestions that conventional antihypertensive strategies based on high dose thiazide therapy had a partial adverse influence on coronary heart disease (9–11), while β-blockers may reduce coronary complications at least in non-smokers (12). On the other hand, it has been postulated that the antihypertensive effect of β-blockers deceases with aging, rendering them less useful as first line agents in the older than in the younger hypertensive population (13). However, this concept was based on a limited number of observations made in a specialized university clinic rather than in a general hypertensive population as it is seen by most practising physicians. The Swiss Bopindolol Study provided an opportunity to assess the relationship between age and the blood pressure (BP)-lowering efficacy of a β-blocker in 622 patients with uncomplicated mild to moderate hypertension treated under usual out-patient conditions.

Methods

Bopindolol is a new β-blocker (14) with slight intrinsic sympathomimetic activity, antihypertensive potency at low dosage (15,16), a long duration of action allowing once daily dosing, and reportedly no relevant influence on serum lipoproteins (17).

The Swiss Bopindolol Study was carried out during a 10-month period in 1984 by a group of practising physicians, who were selected on the basis of their familiarity with the management of hypertensive patients and who were guided by Regional Group Leaders. Preliminary results have been reported recently (18).

The study population included 655 patients (age, 22–80 years) with moderate hypertension, as evidenced by a diastolic BP ranging between 100 and 120 mmHg after a 2-week placebo period and without previous antihypertensive treatment for at least 6 weeks. Patients with retinopathy Keith-Wagener stage III or IV, congestive heart failure, stroke, myocardial infarction within the previous 6 months, serum creatinine $>1\cdot5$ mg/dl, clinical and laboratory evidence for secondary forms of hypertension, patients treated with anti-inflammatory non-steroidal agents, and patients known as 'non-compliant' were excluded. All patients gave their oral consent.

Following the placebo phase (one matched tablet every morning), bopindolol, 1 mg (1 tablet each morning) was given for 12 weeks. Bopindolol dose was decreased to 0·5 mg/day if diastolic BP after 8 weeks was $\leqslant 85$ mmHg; chlorthalidone 12·5 or 25 mg/day was added, if diastolic BP $\geqslant 95$ mmHg after 4 or 8 weeks of bopindolol monotherapy.

The treatment was discontinued early in 33 patients. Complaints promoting the decision to interrupt therapy in 29 patients on bopindolol monotherapy were fatigue ($n=11$), gastrointestinal symptoms ($n=9$), light-headedness ($n=8$), sleeplessness ($n=6$) or vivid dreams ($n=2$), headache ($n=5$), depression ($n=2$), itching and/or skin rash ($n=2$), dyspnea ($n=2$), precordial pain ($n=2$), myalgia ($n=1$) and muscle cramps ($n=1$); in the three patients on combination treatment, gastrointestinal symptoms ($n=1$), dry mouth ($n=1$), light-headedness ($n=1$), muscle cramps ($n=1$)

or impotence ($n = 1$) were reported. Obviously more than one symptom was present in almost all of these patients. In one case uncontrolled hypertension led to interruption of study.

Body weight was measured, blood pressure and heart rate were obtained in the seated position (2 min), and a side-effect questionnaire was completed by the same doctor for a given patient before and after 1 and 2 weeks of the placebo phase and after 4, 8 and 12 weeks of active treatment. Serum potassium (by flame photometer) and creatinine (by autoanalyser) were measured at the same intervals, except for the values after 1 week on placebo.

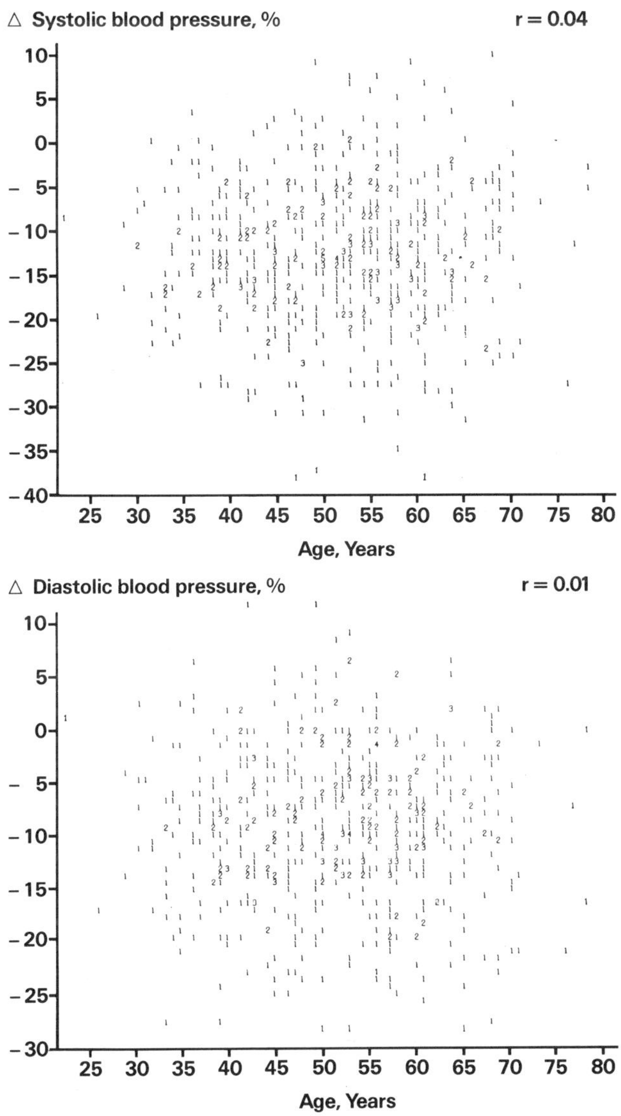

Figure 1. Relationship between age and changes in blood pressure after 4 weeks of bopindolol monotherapy in 622 hypertensive patients. Numbers in the plot denote the number of values on similar co-ordinates.

Statistical analysis of the data was performed by an independent institution (Ulrich Kreuter, PhD, CONSULT AG, Berne, Switzerland). Statistical methods included z-test for comparison of mean values, χ_2 test for analysis of contingency tables, correlation and regression analysis for paired data.

Results

Compared with placebo, blood pressure in the 622 patients completing the study was lowered after 4 weeks of bopindolol monotherapy from 163/106 ± 15/5 to 149/96 ± 17/9 mmHg ($p<0 \cdot 001$). The monotherapy led to a target diastolic BP < 95 mmHg in 302 patients (46%); their blood pressure was decreased from 160/104 ± 14/4 on placebo to 141/90 ± 13/6 mmHg after 4 weeks and remained at 139/89 ± 13/6 mmHg at 12 weeks of bopindolol monotherapy.

In 320 patients, blood pressure was not controlled after 4 weeks of bopindolol monotherapy (156/102 ± 17/7 as compared with 166/106 ± 16/6 mmHg on placebo); the addition of chlorthalidone lowered blood pressure ($p<0 \cdot 001$) to 145/95 ± 15/7 mmHg at 12 weeks and achieved target diastolic BP > 95 mmHg in 167 patients (25% of total population).

Absolute or percentage decreases in blood pressure induced by bopindolol monotherapy did not correlate with age (Fig. 1). Moreover, age as well as body weight, heart rate and serum creatinine obtained on placebo conditions were on average similar in patients responding to monotherapy as compared with those requiring combination therapy (Table 1). The latter differed from the monotherapy group by a higher initial blood pressure ($p<0 \cdot 001$) and a lower female/male ratio.

During active treatment, heart rate was decreased ($p<0 \cdot 0001$) similarly in the two groups (−9 beats/min). Body weight and serum creatinine were largely unchanged. Serum potassium was not significantly changed during β-blocker monotherapy (4·34 ± 0·41 to 4·41 ± 0·43 mmol/l and decreased minimally during combination treatment (4·37 ± 0·45 to 4·00 ± 0·45 mmol/l).

Discussion

In this study population of 655 patients with moderate hypertension, the mean age (51 years) and distribution of sex (46% women, 53% men) were quite similar to characteristics of the average hypertensive population. Bopindolol alone or combined with low dose chlorthalidone provided a satisfactory blood pressure reduction in 71% of the study population. This response rate corresponds well with that obtained previously with other β-blockers prescribed alone or in combination with diuretics (19).

The main finding of the present study is that β-blocker-induced absolute or percentage blood pressure-reductions were unrelated to age ($r=0 \cdot 07$ to $0 \cdot 10$), which in this large study population ranged from 22 to 80 years. Moreover, the mean age in the group responding to β-blocker monotherapy and those requiring the addition of a diuretic was similar in the present and a previous study (19).

These observations militate against an age-related antihypertensive efficacy of β-blockers (13), including bopindolol (15), a claim derived from considerably smaller groups of subjects studied in the selection-prone setting of a specialized university clinic rather than in a hypertensive population seen in general practice. It is concluded

Table 1

Findings under placebo conditions in the 655 patients (mean ± SD).

	Patients completing study			'Drop-outs'
	Receiving bopindolol monotherapy	Receiving combination therapy	All	
n	302	320	622	33
Age (years)	15·5 ± 10·0	51·5 ± 9·9	51·5 ± 10·0	51·5 ± 10·0
Female/male	154/148	140/180	294/328	14/19
Body weight (kg)	76·3 ± 13·7	77·7 ± 13·9	77·0 ± 13·8	76·2 ± 15·0
Blood pressure (mmHg)[a,b]	160/104 ± 14/5	166/108 ± 16/6[c]	163/106 ± 15/5	162/107 ± 17/6
Heart rate, beats/min[a,b]	76 ± 9	78/10	77 ± 10	74 ± 9
Serum creatinine, mg/dl	1·0 ± 0·2	1·0 ± 0·2	1·0 ± 0·2	1·1 ± 0·2

[a]Obtained in the seated position; [b]Mean of values after 1 and 2 weeks placebo; [c]$p < 0{\cdot}001$ vs monotherapy group.

that age is not a relevant determinant of the potency of bopindolol and perhaps also other β-blockers in practical antihypertensive treatment. With consideration of the usual contraindications, bopindolol is a useful β-blocker for the treatment of various age groups with hypertension.

Acknowledgements

The authors would like to thank all the practising physicians and regional group leaders who aided in this study.

Group leaders included Drs Hans Albert, Winterthur; Walter Angehrn, St Gallen; O. Bass, Biel; J. P. Berger, Vevey; H. Biedermann, Münsterlingen; A. Blumberg, Aarau; H. R. Brunner, Lausanne; H. J. Bucher, Luzern; F. Bühler, Basel; J. P. Bussien, Lausanne; P. Cottier, Interlaken; P. M. Dufour, Sion; J. F. Enrico, Neuchâtel; H. J. Gloor, Schaffhausen; A. Grandchamp, Genève; G. Keusch, Zürich; A. Koelz, Liestal; J. Ludin, Olten; G. A. Lupi, Solothurn; T. Moccetti, Lugano; A. Nanzer, Visp; M. Pajarola, Chur; M. Périat, Porrentruy; V. Ruiz, Fribourg; A. de Torrenté, La Chaux-de-Fonds; W. Vetter, Zürich; Jakob Wanner, Rüti; P. Weidmann, Chairman, Bern.

The authors also acknowledge the expert statistical analysis by Ulrich Kreuter, PhD, Consult AG, Bern.

References

(1) Waal-Manning HJ. Hypertension: which betablocker? *Drugs* 1976; **12**: 312–441.

(2) Wilcox RG. Randomized study of six betablockers and a thiazide diuretic in essential hypertension. *Br Med J* 1978; **2**: 383–385.

(3) Weidmann P, Fuss O. Medikamentöse Hypertoniebehandlung 1977. Empirische und rationale Gesichtspunkte. *Schweiz Med Wschr* 1978; **108**: 1–18.

(4) Medical Research Council Working Party on Mild to Moderate Hypertension. Adverse reactions to bendrofluazide and propranolol for the treatment of mild hypertension. *Lancet* 1981; **ii**: 539–543.

(5) Murphy MB, Lewis PJ, Kohner E, Schumer B, Dollery CT. Glucose intolerance in hypertensive patients treated with diuretics; a fourteen year follow-up. *Lancet* 1982; **ii**: 1293–1295.

(6) Weidmann P, Gerber A, Mordasini R. Effects of antihypertensive therapy on serum lipoproteins. *Hypertension* 1982; **5**(suppl III): III120–III131.

(7) Kaplan NM. Our appropriate concern about hypokalemia. *Am J Med* 1984; **77**: 1–4.

(8) Struthers AD, Murphy MB, Dollery CT. Glucose tolerance during antihypertensive therapy in patients with diabetes mellitus. *Hypertension* 1985; **7**(suppl II): II95–II101.

(9) Helgeland A. Treatment of mild hypertension: a five year controlled drug trial. The Oslo Study. *Am J Med* 1980; **69**; 725–732.

(10) Morgan TO, Adams WR, Hodgson M, Gibberd RW. Failure of therapy to improve prognosis in elderly males with hypertension. *Med J Aust* 1980; **2**: 27–31.

(11) Multiple Risk Factor Intervention Trial. Risk factor changes and mortality results. *JAMA* 1982; **248**: 1465–1477.

(12) Medical Research Council Working Party: MRC trial of treatment of mild hypertension: Principal results. *Br Med J* 1985; **291**: 97–104.

(13) Bühler FR, Burkart F, Lütold BE, Küng M, Marbet G, Pfisterer M. Antihypertensive beta blocking action as related to renin and age: A pharmacological tool to identify pathogenetic mechanism in essential hypertension. *Am J Cardiol* 1975; **36**: 653–669.

(14) Aellig WH. Pharmacological experiments in healthy volunteers with bopindolol, a long-acting β-adrenoceptor blocking drug with partial agonist activity. *Br J Clin Pharmacol* 1985; **19**: 775–781.

(15) Hulthén UL, van Brummelen P, Amann FW, Bühler FR. Antihypertensive efficacy of the new long-acting betablocker bopindolol as related to age. *J Cardiovasc Pharmacol* 1983; **5**: 426–492.

(16) Andersson O, Hedner T, Nyberg G. Long-term antihypertensive effects of bopindolol once daily or once weekly. *Eur J Clin Pharmacol* 1985; (in press).

(17) van Brummelen P, Bolli P, Koolen MI, Staehelin HB, Bühler FR. Plasma lipid fractions during long-term monotherapy with the ISA-containing beta-adrenoceptor blocker bopindolol in hypertensive patients. *Br J Clin Pharmacol* 1984; **17**: 86–88.

(18) Weidmann P, Bousquet J-Ch and the Swiss Practitioners Bopindolol Study Group. Antihypertensive treatment with bopindolol alone or combined with a diuretic in general practice. *J Cardiovasc Pharmacol* 1985 (in press).

(19) Veterans Administration Cooperative Study Group on Antihypertensive Agents. Propranolol in the treatment of essential hypertension. *JAMA* 1977; **237**: 2303–2310.

Bopindolol vs metoprolol in hypertension: comparison of clinical efficacy and tolerance in a double-blind, parallel study

R. F. WESTERMAN,[1] C. CHRISTENSEN,[2] A. WESTHEIM,[2] and A. J. M. DONKER[1]

[1]*Department of Medicine, Free University Hospital, Amsterdam, The Netherlands*
[2]*Clinic for Cardiology and Medicine, Oslo, Norway*

Introduction

β-Adrenergic receptor antagonists have achieved and maintain an established position in the treatment of hypertension. They all lower blood pressure to a similar degree. Differences in secondary characteristics such as presence or absence of intrinsic sympathomimetic activity (ISA), duration of action and specificity for β-1 receptors (incorrectly called 'cardioselectivity'). Bopindolol is a non-specific β-adrenergic receptor antagonist with mild intrinsic sympathomimetic activity (1). It has a long duration of action. A single oral dose showed to inhibit exercise-induced tachycardia for over 24 h (2). This suggests bopindolol once daily being useful in the treatment of hypertension without a need for a slow release formulation (3,4,5). Even a once weekly regimen gave satisfactory results (6).

The present study was planned in order to examine the usefulness of bopindolol in comparison to the established β-blocker metoprolol in the treatment of hypertension. Earlier comparisons with propranolol (5) and atenolol (7) have already been performed as well as with metoprolol (6).

Andersson studied 14 patients with initial diastolic pressures between 95 and 125 mmHg and systolic pressures such that mean arterial pressure was >117 mmHg for those aged 30–39 and >127 for those of 40–59 years. In a double-blind, crossover study bopindolol 1–2 mg daily was compared with metoprolol 100–200 mg daily. The periods were an open run-in period (no treatment over 4 weeks), a placebo wash-out (single-blind for 4 weeks) and 6 weeks double-blind bopindolol or metoprolol treatment. With both drugs and in both supine and standing positions reductions in blood pressure and heart rate were comparable and highly significant.

The position of bopindolol, a new β-blocker, edited by P. A. van Zwieten, 1987: Royal Society of Medicine Services International Congress and Symposium Series No. 106, published by Royal Society of Medicine Services Limited.

In our study the aims were to compare clinical efficacy as well as clinical and laboratory tolerance in patients with moderate and severe hypertension.

Patients and methods

The study was performed with an identical protocol independently in Oslo and Amsterdam without the doctors having contact. Accordingly, the results were analysed independently. Subsequently, combined results were processed.

Bopindolol and metoprolol were studied double-blind in parallel groups of patients after random allocation of the drugs to the patients.

Patients

Eligible for the study were out-patients of both sexes between 20 and 60 years of age with a diagnosis of essential hypertension and having a diastolic blood pressure (seated) between 105 and 120 mmHg at the end of a placebo period of 3 weeks. Blood pressure was measured with the London School of Hygiene and Tropical Medicine Sphygmomanometer. Measurements were taken before 10 h 00 and prior to the morning drug dosage. Excluded were patients with contraindications for β-blocker therapy (asthma, heart failure), concomitant illnesses interfering with a proper assessment of the results (liver, renal or gastrointestinal disease), the likelihood of early pregnancy and non-compliant patients. Twenty-four patients were expected to complete the study in each centre.

Drugs

Bopindolol was dispensed in capsules of 2 mg, metoprolol in capsules of 100 mg.

Patients commenced with a 3-week placebo period. Subsequently, they were randomized to treatment with fixed dosage of either 2 mg bopindolol once daily or 100 mg metoprolol twice daily. After completion of 3 weeks' therapy active treatment was either continued for a further 3-week period at the same dosage or the dosage was increased to a fixed double dosage, depending on the achievement of diastolic pressure to $\leqslant$90 mmHg or not. Active treatment lasted for 9 weeks.

Dosage schedule

The placebo period was a maximum of 3 weeks: 2 × 1 capsules of placebo were given daily.

Dose finding and therapy period (9 weeks)

First phase of 3 weeks. One capsule of bopindolol (2 μg) was given in the morning and one capsule of placebo in the evening, or 2 × 1 capsule of metoprolol (2 × 100 mg).

Second phase of 3 weeks. If necessary the dosage was increased to two capsules of bopindolol (4 mg) in the morning and two capsules of placebo in the evening, or 2×2 capsules of metoprolol (2×200 mg).

Third phase of 3 weeks. If necessary, additional therapy such as a peripheral vasodilator was given.

Efficacy was judged by systolic and diastolic blood pressures; tolerance and safety by heart rate, side-effects, ECG and laboratory results.

Statistical evaluation

For changes in blood pressure and pulse rate Wilcoxon's signed rank test ($2\alpha = 0 \cdot 05$) was used to compare effects with baseline pressures per treatment group. Comparisons between groups were performed by using the U-test (Mann-Whitney-Wilcoxon). In the tables of results data are shown as means ±SD.

Results

Patients

In Amsterdam the required diastolic pressure above 105 mmHg at the end of the placebo period was measured in 16 patients. In Oslo 23 patients entered the study but three had to be removed from the study due to side-effects. No other drop-outs were observed in either city.

After decoding the patients appeared to be allocated as shown in Table 1.

Patients in Oslo were somewhat older and more overweight than those in Amsterdam. One patient in each of the Amsterdam treatment groups had a diastolic pressure above 120 mmHg but none were below 105 mmHg. Systolic values were in all cases above normal (140 mmHg), but in most cases only moderately elevated. Accordingly, the patients studied in Amsterdam had predominantly diastolic hypertension. Oslo patients had higher systolic pressures on average.

Table 1

	Bopindolol	Metoprolol
Amsterdam		
male/female	3/4	4/5
mean age years (range)	45 (24–63)	46 (35–58)
mean weight kg (range)	75 (54–94)	75 (59–88)
mean height cm (range)	168 (142–177)	166 (157–179)
Oslo		
male/female	8/4	8/3
mean age years (range)	55 (40–65)	52 (37–60)
mean weight kg (range)	81 (63–112)	88 (72–115)
mean height cm (range)	172 (158–188)	174 (158–188)

Dosage after 9 weeks of treatment

In Amsterdam bopindolol dosage after 9 weeks was 2 mg daily in one patient and 4 mg in six patients; the dosage of metoprolol was 400 mg daily in all nine patients who used this drug. In Oslo bopindolol dosage after 9 weeks was 2 mg daily in four patients and 4 mg in six; the dosage of metoprolol was 200 mg in two patients, 400 mg in eight.

Effect on blood pressure

Results are summarized in Table 2.

In Amsterdam after the placebo period systolic blood pressure showed a significant difference between the two groups (bopindolol group 156 mmHg; metoprolol group 168 mmHg), implying that distribution of baseline values for systolic blood pressure was not homogeneous ($p=0\cdot034$). Both systolic and diastolic blood pressure decreased significantly at a 5% level during treatment. No statistically significant differences could be demonstrated between the two treatments.

In Oslo, at the end of the placebo period, systolic and diastolic pressures did not differ significantly from each other in the two treatment groups but at the end of the trial a significant difference in efficacy of treatment became apparent. Diastolic blood pressure was reduced −9 mmHg in the bopindolol group and −15 mmHg in the metoprolol group ($p=0\cdot045$). Calculations on the combined data from both cities again showed significant reductions in blood pressure during treatment. Between the two treatment groups the difference were statistically not significant.

Normalization of blood pressure

In Amsterdam after 9 weeks of treatment two patients in the bopindolol group had achieved a 'normal' diastolic pressure (= <90 mmHg) against one in the metoprolol treated group.

In Oslo after 9 weeks of treatment two patients came under 90 mmHg diastolic in the bopindolol group against four in the metoprolol group.

The responder rate with bopindolol was 83% in Oslo and 86% in Amsterdam and with metoprolol in Oslo 73% and in Amsterdam 78% (the degree of response was calculated as the percentage reduction in the excess of the mean arterial pressure over the normal value for the patient's age being 107 mmHg < 30 years and 117 mmHg > = 30 years; the responder rate was defined as the percentage of patients in whom this reduction equalled or exceeded 50%.

The normalization rate was 25% with bopindolol in Oslo and 43% in Amsterdam. With metoprolol it was 55% in Oslo and 11% in Amsterdam (normalization rate was defined as the percentage of patients achieving a blood pressure of 140 mmHg systolic *and* 90 mmHg diastolic if age below 30 years, or 160 mmHg *and* 95 mmHg diastolic if age 30 years or over).

Heart rate in Amsterdam was more reduced with metoprolol than with bopindolol ($p=0\cdot095$). The average values are shown in Table 3. In Oslo, heart rate did not differ in either group. For the combined results for bopindolol it was 78 ± 16 (initial) and 64 ± 9 (9 weeks) and for metoprolol 78 ± 12 (initial) and 60 ± 10 (9 weeks). Again this implied no difference between the two drugs.

Table 2

Blood pressure changes with bopindolol and metoprolol

	Amsterdam			Oslo			Combined		
	initial	3 weeks	9 weeks	initial	3 weeks	9 weeks	initial	3 weeks	9 weeks
Bopindolol									
systolic	156 ± 8	148 ± 12*	144 ± 13*	161 ± 17	143 ± 19***	146 ± 21**	159 ± 16	145 ± 16	146 ± 17**
diastolic	112 ± 5	98 ± 7*	95 ± 9*	105 ± 4	94 ± 11*	98 ± 9*	109 ± 6	98 ± 7***	96 ± 9***
Metoprolol									
systolic	168 ± 11	155 ± 17*	159 ± 20*	164 ± 19*	150 ± 35*	147 ± 33*	165 ± 15	152 ± 28**	152 ± 30*
diastolic	115 ± 9	104 ± 7*	101 ± 11*	110 ± 5	97 ± 11**	94 ± 15**	112 ± 8	100 ± 10**	97 ± 14***

$^{*}p = <0{\cdot}05$; $^{**}p = <0{\cdot}01$; $^{***}p = <0{\cdot}001$

Table 3
Pulse rate changes during treatment

	Amsterdam		Oslo		Combined	
	initial	9 weeks	initial	9 weeks	initial	9 weeks
Bopindolol	76 ± 13	67 ± 11*	77 ± 19	63 ± 8*	78 ± 16	64 ± 9*
Metoprolol	79 ± 14	57 ± 9*	77 ± 12	62 ± 10*	78 ± 12	60 ± 10*

*$p = < 0{\cdot}05$

Side effects

In Amsterdam three of the seven patients in the bopindolol group complained of a total of four side-effects compared with eight of the nine patients in the metoprolol group who reported a total of nine different side-effects. In Oslo seven patients treated with bopindolol complained 14 times of 10 different side-effects against three patients treated with metoprolol who reported five times four different side-effects.

Together, the list shown in Table 4 was compiled:

Table 4

	Bopindolol	Metoprolol
Sleep disturbances	3	3
Drowsiness	1	—
Fatigue	1	1
Headache	1	3
Dizziness, vertigo	4	2
Restlessness	1	—
Blurred vision	—	1
Tightness in chest	1	2
Dry or painful eyes	1	2
Nausea, indigestion, dyspepsia	3	1
Cold feet	—	1
Pain in the legs	1	—
Weakness in the legs	—	1
Nocturia	1	1

In Amsterdam none of the patients had to interrupt treatment because of side-effects. One patient developed a psychoneurosis and was withdrawn from the studies after 6 weeks. In Oslo three patients interrupted treatment because of side-effects, two patients with bopindolol (2 mg) and one patient with metoprolol (100 mg).

Eye examination

In Amsterdam five of the six patients in the bopindolol group who completed the study were examined before and after the study as well as five of the nine patients in the metoprolol group. In no case evidence for an oculo-muco-cutaneous syndrome was found. This also counted for the patient in the metoprolol group who complained of dry and burning eyes during the first few weeks of treatment. In Oslo nine out of 12 patients in the bopindolol group were seen by the ophthalmologist and 10 of the 11 in the metoprolol group. Also here an oculo-muco-cutaneous syndrome did not appear.

Laboratory results

During the study no clinically relevant changes were observed in haemoglobin, total and differential WBC, and serum sodium, potassium, creatinine, uric acid, urea, gamma-GT, ASAT and ALAT.

Discussion

The results of this study show that bopindolol is an effective and well-tolerated blood pressure lowering agent. This is in accordance with earlier observations (3–7). Reduction in blood pressure was comparable to that obtained with metoprolol. Whereas blood pressure measurements were taken before administration of the morning dose, it appears that once daily bopindolol is as effective as twice daily metoprolol in reducing blood pressure with a similar pattern and incidence of side-effects. The long duration of action may make this drug attractive if dosage of a lower frequency than once daily is preferred. This may be an important characteristics of this β-blocker.

The doses chosen in this study were rather well-matched. The bopindolol doses of 2 and 4 mg daily were comparable to the metoprolol doses of 200 and 400 mg daily in their effects. Now that the blood pressure lowering effect of bopindolol has been compared with that of propranolol (5), metoprolol (6) and atenolol (7), further experience will teach us whether important differences in side-effects will occur between these drugs during prolonged use.

Acknowledgement

Materials and technical and statistical assistance were kindly provided by Sandoz, Basle, Switzerland.

References

(1) Berthold R, Waite R, Weber H. Pharmacological studies with bopindolol: a new long-acting beta-adrenoceptor antagonist (Abstract). *Brit J Pharmacol* 1981; **74**: 829.

(2) Aellig WH. Pharmacological experiments in healthy volunteers with bopindolol, a long-acting β-adrenoceptor blocking drug with partial agonist activity. *Br J Clin Pharmacol* 1985; **19**: 775–781.

(3) van Brummelen P, Bühler FR, Ammann FW, Bolli P. Effects of a new long-acting beta-blocker bopindolol (LT 31-200) on blood pressure, plasma catecholamines, renin and cholesterol in patients with arterial hypertension. *Eur J Clin Pharmacol* 1982; **22**: 491–493.

(4) Hulthén UL, van Brummelen P, Ammann FW, Bühler FR. Antihypertensive efficacy of the new long-acting beta-blocker bopindolol as related to age. *J Cardiovasc Pharmacol* 1983; **5**: 426.
(5) Kirch W, Axthelm T. Bopindolol, a new long-acting beta-adrenoceptor antagonist—a randomized comparison against propranolol in hypertensive patients. *Int J Clin Pharmacol Res* 1983; **3**: 89–93.
(6) Andersson OK, Hedner T, Nyberg G. Acute and long-term antihypertensive effect of bopindolol—a nonselective beta-adrenergic blocker with ISA. *Eur J Clin Pharmacol* 1985; **29**: 281–285.
(7) Abétel G, Mérier G, Karly M, Genoud A, Bousquet JC. Intérèt du profil tensionnel dans l'evaluation de deux antihypertenseurs. *Schweiz Med Wschr* 1984; **114**: 1746–1749.

Bopindolol vs metoprolol in patients with hypertension and a left ventricular ejection fraction less than 55%

SIMON H. BRAAT, ANTON P. M. GORGELS and EUGÈNE HARDY

University Hospital of Maastricht, University of Limburg, Maastricht, The Netherlands

Summary

A double-blind study was undertaken to compare the effects of bopindolol, a new β-blocking agent, given once daily with metoprolol, given twice daily, on blood pressure and left ventricular ejection fraction.

The inclusion criteria of a diastolic blood pressure above 95 mmHg and a left ventricular ejection fraction below 55% were fulfilled by 18 patients.

A lowering of the diastolic blood pressure below a value of 95 mmHg was achieved after treatment with bopindolol or metoprolol in all patients. In both groups a significant decrease in heart rate was observed but no significant change in left ventricular ejection fraction occurred.

We concluded that bopindolol as well as metoprolol reduce diastolic blood pressure; both drugs cause a significant lowering of the heart rate and do not lead to a significant effect on left ventricular ejection fraction.

Introduction

β-adrenergic blocking drugs have long been a cornerstone in the medical management of hypertension. Although well tolerated by most patients many clinicians are reluctant to use these drugs in patients with depressed left ventricular function because of their negative inotropic and chronotropic properties.

Bopindolol (LT 31-200) is a new, long acting, non-selective β-adrenoceptor antagonist with modest intrinsic sympathomimetic activity (ISA) (1). It was the aim of the present study to compare bopindolol vs metoprolol in regard to clinical efficacy and safety in patients with hypertension and depressed left ventricular function.

The position of bopindolol, a new β-blocker, edited by P. A. van Zwieten, 1987: Royal Society of Medicine Services International Congress and Symposium Series No. 106, published by Royal Society of Medicine Services Limited.

Patients and methods

A randomized double-blind parallel group study design was used after a placebo 'wash-out' period of 1–3 weeks; patients were allocated to either bopindolol or metoprolol at random. In the placebo period all previous antihypertensive treatment was omitted. The inclusion criteria for the study were male or female patients aged below 70 years, with moderate or severe essential hypertension. The diastolic blood pressure had to be at least above 105 mmHg at the end of the placebo period and a left ventricular ejection fraction (LVEF) measured with radionuclide techniques of less than 55%. (Normal value in our laboratory is ≥60%) (2). Exclusion criteria were: cardiac failure, pulmonary disease, liver or renal impairment, diabetes mellitus requiring insulin and pregnant or lactating women.

In the placebo phase all patients received a placebo capsule in the morning and one in the evening. At the end of this period the following investigations were performed. A nuclear angiogram to be able to calculate the left ventricular ejection fraction; a chest X-ray, laboratory tests: haemoglobin, total white blood cells sedimentation rate, urea, creatinine, glucose, transaminases and an electrocardiogram. During the first 2 weeks of the treatment period the patients received 1 mg of bopindolol in the morning and a placebo in the evening or 50 mg of metoprolol in the morning and the evening.

All drugs were given by mouth. The aim of treatment was to achieve a diastolic blood pressure of less than 95 mmHg and the dosage was doubled after 3 and 6 weeks if this goal was not achieved. The maximum dose of bopindolol was 4 mg daily and of metoprolol 200 mg twice daily. If the blood pressure did not drop below the target level of 95 mmHg with this maximal dose a vasodilator had to be added to the therapy.

Blood pressure was recorded with the patients sitting after 5 min rest, the diastolic being taken when the sounds were muffled (Korotkoff IV). Tolerance was assessed by recording information on side-effects and safety by clinical examinations and ECG and clinical history at all visits.

When the goal of the treatment was achieved laboratory data were obtained again and a second nuclear angiogram was made to calculate the LVEF during treatment.

Changes in left ventricular ejection fraction during the course of the study were analysed using the paired student-t-test.

Results

Eighteen patients were included in the study: 11 were males, age varied between 35–68 years with a mean of 54 years. Nine of them received Metoprolol and nine bopindolol. Of the nine patients treated with bopindolol, two patients achieved a diastolic blood pressure below 95 mmHg with 1 mg bopindolol, four patients with 2 mg and two patients with 4 mg. One patient refused all medication after 6 weeks because of restlessness. In the metoprolol treated group four patients achieved a diastolic blood pressure below 95 mmHg with 2×50 mg, and five patients with 2×100 mg.

The left ventricular ejection fraction in the patients treated with bopindolol varied in the placebo phase between 42 and 55% (mean 50 ± 4%) and during the treatment with a dose of bopindolol, which had caused a drop in the diastolic blood pressure below 95 mmHg between 42 and 65% (mean 53 ± 7%). This difference was not statistically significant.

In the group of patients treated with metoprolol the left ventricular ejection fraction in the placebo phase varied between 48 and 55% (mean $51 \pm 3\%$) and in the period in which the patients were treated with metoprolol between 42 and 65% (mean $55 \pm 9\%$). This difference is not statistically significant. The heart rate in the placebo phase of the patients treated with bopindolol varied between 70 and 130 beats/min (mean 88 ± 21) and during the treatment with bopindolol between 50 and 100 beats/min (mean 69 ± 14). This difference is statistically significant ($p < 0{\cdot}02$).

The heart rate in the placebo phase of the patients later treated with metoprolol varied between 70 and 105 beats/min (mean 80 ± 14) and during treatment between 55 and 100 beats/min (mean 69 ± 13). This difference is statistically significant ($p < 0{\cdot}01$).

Except for one patient in the bopindolol group who dropped out because of restlessness the side-effects were mild and no abnormalities were noticed in the laboratory data.

Discussion

β-Adrenergic blocking agents decrease heart rate and cardiac output and increase left ventricular volume (3–4). These effects are weaker or absent for β-blockers with ISA. The decrease in cardiac output has been primarily attributed to a reduction in heart rate, but may also be related to depression of myocardial contractility. Since bopindolol is a new long-acting non-selective β-adrenoceptor antagonist with ISA, one would expect a smaller drop in heart rate compared to patients treated with β-blocking agents without ISA and therefore also a smaller decrease of cardiac output. In patients with an impaired left ventricular function, who are treated with β-blocking agents, one would prefer on theoretical grounds a β-blocking agent with significant ISA.

In our study, however, we did not find any significant worsening of the left ventricular dysfunction in the patients treated with bopindolol or metoprolol.

Accordingly, we conclude that in patients with hypertension and a left ventricular dysfunction β-blocking agents can be used with relative safety.

References

(1) Berthold R, Waite R, Weber H. Pharmacological studies with bopindolol: a new long action beta adrenoceptor antagonist. (Abstract). *Br J Pharmacol* 1982; **74**: 829 P.

(2) Braat SH, Brugada P, Zwaan de C, Den Dulk K, Wellens HJJ. Right and left ventricular ejection fraction in acute inferior wall infarction with or without ST segment elevation in V4R. *JACC* 1984; **4**: 940–944.

(3) Hamer J. Beta adrenergic blocking drugs. In: Hamer J, ed. *Drugs for heart disease*. Chicago: Year Book Medical Publishers, 1979: 148–243.

(4) Gibson DG. Pharmacodynamic properties of beta adrenergic receptor blocking drugs in man. *Drugs* 1974; **7**: 8–38.

Efficacy of bopindolol, a new β-blocking agent in angina pectoris compared to metoprolol

AART VERMEULEN

Andreas Hospital, Amsterdam, The Netherlands

Summary

Bopindolol is a recently developed, non-specific β-adrenoreceptor antagonist with a prolonged duration of action and sympathomimetic activity.

Fifteen patients with stable angina pectoris (class 2/4 NYHA) were selected. Four patients had insufficient anginal attacks during the placebo-phase and one patient developed unstable angina pectoris. Ten patients were randomized to either bopindolol (1–4 mg/day) ($n = 5$) or metoprolol (100–400 mg/day) ($n = 5$).

Both medicaments were equally effective in lowering the frequency and the severity of anginal attacks, with a decreased consumption of nitroglycerine. None of the patients treated with bopindolol and two patients treated with metoprolol complained of side-effects (dizziness).

Sandonorm, in a once daily dose, is as at least effective in treating angina pectoris as a metoprolol, twice daily, and there is a tendency to fewer side-effects.

Introduction

To evaluate bopindolol, a new β-receptor antagonist, with respect to its efficacy for treatment of patients with angina pectoris, a study was undertaken to compare its effects with metoprolol, a widely used β_1-selective β-receptor antagonist. Bopindolol has no selectivity for β-receptors but at least in animal models shows some intrinsic sympathomimetic activity (ISA). The advantages advocated are the low dose necessary to reach a therapeutic effect and the long half-life which makes it possible to prescribe the medication once daily, also in angina pectoris.

The position of bopindolol, a new β-blocker, edited by P. A. van Zwieten, 1987: Royal Society of Medicine Services International Congress and Symposium Series No. 106, published by Royal Society of Medicine Services Limited.

Design of the study

Patients started with tapering off their original medication in the course of 1 week. After a 2–4 week single-blind placebo period patients, who met the entrance criteria (i.e. at least three exercise induced anginal attacks a week for the last 2 weeks of placebo), were randomly allocated to either treatment with bopindolol or metoprolol. Patients were seen after 4 weeks and the dose of the medication was adjusted if necessary.

At each visit the diary was controlled, a physical examination was made, a resting ECG, blood tests were performed at the end of the placebo phase and after 4 and 12 weeks of active treatment.

Patient material

Fifteen patients with a documented diagnosis of coronary artery disease (a positive exercise test and/or 50% stenosis out the coronary angiogram) and angina pectoris and normal tension were selected for the study.

Five patients dropped out, one because of rapid deterioration of his angina pectoris after which he decided to restart his former medication, the other four did not reach the entry criteria at the end of the placebo period. Ten patients were randomised; five for treatment with bopindolol and five for medication with metoprolol.

The two groups did not differ in age, weight, height, blood pressure and nitroglycerine consumption (Table 1).

Table 1

Patients treated with either bopindolol or metoprolol

		Bopindolol	Metoprolol
Sex	male	4	3
	female	1	2
Age (years		60·8 ± 9·8	62·8 ± 10·1
Weight (kg)		77 ± 10·2	73 ± 10·2
Height (cm)		167 ± 5·9	171 ± 10·9
Blood pressure		139/83	147/86
Nitroglycerine consumption (mg/week)		4·72 ± 4·68	3·67 ± 2·79

Anginal attacks

The number and severity of attacks were recorded by the patients on diary cards, and the weekly number of attacks was registered.

The effect of treatment on anginal attacks was assessed by means of the angina index:

$$(\text{number of mild attacks} \times 1) + (\text{number of moderate attacks} \times 2) + (\text{number of severe attacks} \times 3)$$

Results

The anginal score decreased in both groups (Table 3, Wilcoxon sum rank test $p<0 \cdot 01$) as did the nitroglycerine consumption (Table 4). There were no changes in blood chemistry, no signs of cardiac failure, and no ECG-changes. None of the patients treated with bopindolol and two patients treated with metoprolol complained of subjective side-effects (dizziness).

Heart rate at rest was lowered by both metoprolol and bopindolol (Table 2).

The resting blood pressure remained unchanged during treatment with either of the two β-blockers.

Table 2

The effect of β-blocker medication on resting heart rate

	Heart rate at rest (end placebo)	Heart rate at rest after 12 weeks treatment
Bopindolol	78·2±12·0	62·2±7·6
Metoprolol	71·4±8·3	56·2±9·7

Table 3

Weekly sum of anginal attack score per patient during 4 weeks placebo and 4 weeks active therapy at the end of the study period.

Angina score	Period I				Period IV			
Bopindolol								
1	20	15	23	7	5	0	1	6
8	11	35			5	3	5	0
11	8	6	6	11	1	0	2	2
12	4	2	2	5	0	0	0	1
14	5	4	4	5	2	0	2	2
Metoprolol								
2	6	10	12	8	10	12	8	12
3	12	11	20	18	13	10	7	8
5	20	42	19	21	8	4	3	2
9	26	13	17	9	5	3	5	10
15	1	6	4	9	11	6	2	2

Table 4

Weekly consumption of nitroglycerine (mg) during the placebo period and during the last 4 weeks of the active treatment

	Period I	Period IV
Bopindolol	4·72±4·68	1·02±0·99
Metoprolol	3·67±2·79	2·42±1·62

Discussion

The beneficial effect of β-adrenoceptor antagonists in angina pectoris is widely recognized. However, little is known about the details of the pathophysiological mechanism of this therapeutic effect. It is assumed that the lowering of the workload of the heart due to both the reduction in heart rate and systolic blood pressure during exercise, are major factors in postponing attacks of angina pectoris.

All types of β-adrenoceptor antagonists appear to display beneficial effects, thus the difference between different substances must be sought in their total action on the cardiovascular system. The side-effects induced by the increase in peripheral resistance i.e. cold extremities are less important for drugs with ISA.

However, in the present study no difference was observed between metoprolol and bopindolol. The long duration of action of bopindolol was obvious also in the present study, where a once daily dose proved effective in the treatment of angina. However, no data are available concerning the time-related effect on exercise induced angina pectoris.

Conclusions

In a small series of patients, bopindolol decreased the frequency of exercise-induced angina pectoris in a once daily dosage. Exercise testing in a larger group of patients should be performed to establish the exact effect of bopindolol compared with that of other β-receptor antagonists.

Conclusions: the profile of bopindolol

P. A. VAN ZWIETEN

Division of Pharmacotherapy, Faculty of Medicine, University of Amsterdam, Amsterdam, The Netherlands

General conclusions

It was the aim of the present symposium to establish, as far as possible, the pharmacological and clinical characteristics of bopindolol, as well as comparing it with the impressive number of β-blockers now available. The following conclusions and opinions were established in concensus by the participants of the round table conference.

Receptor profile and potency

Bopindolol is a non-selective $\beta_1 + \beta_2$-adrenoceptor blocking drug, as established in all *in vitro* animal and human studies. A moderate degree of intrinsic sympathomimetic activity (ISA), though weaker than that of pindolol or oxprenolol, could be demonstrated *in vitro* (spontaneously beating isolated atria from reserpinized rats). In addition, the reduction of β_2-adrenoceptor density on lymphocytes in healthy volunteers treated with bopindolol is also in concordance with the profile of a non-selective β-blocker with some ISA. The reduction of β_2-receptor density would point towards a reduced tendency to evoke withdrawal phenomena upon sudden interruption of treatment, in particular in patients with angina, as observed for other β-blockers with ISA.

However, in clinical studies on haemodynamics (see below) the ISA of bopindolol cannot always be demonstrated and remains subject to debate.

In all animal and human models bopindolol appears to be the most potent β-adrenoceptor blocking drug so far available. This high potency is reflected by its low oral dosage (1–2 mg daily) when used in the treatment of essential hypertension.

Haemodynamic profile

In chronic studies with human hypertensives bopindolol induced a fall in blood pressure, heart rate and cardiac output, whereas stroke volume remained virtually

The position of bopindolol, a new β-blocker, edited by P. A. van Zwieten, 1987: Royal Society of Medicine Services International Congress and Symposium Series No. 106, published by Royal Society of Medicine Services Limited.

unchanged. Total peripheral resistance (TPR) only rose during the first few hours when bopindolol was given orally (2 mg), to reach baseline values after a few hours. Upon chronic treatment TPR remained unchanged. This profile points towards effective, potent β-adrenoceptor blockade, although ISA could not be demonstrated convincingly, a fact which seems to agree with current knowledge that drugs with potent ISA are known to significantly reduce TPR.

In circadian studies, β-blockers with ISA are known to increase heart rate during the night and hence to prevent its naturally occurring decrease. In human hypertensives or patients with coronary heart disease treated with bopindolol, heart rate during the night remained the same as in the control period, whereas atenolol, a drug devoid of ISA, reduced heart rate both during the day and at night. These findings suggest that bopindolol would possess weak ISA. A possible influence of bopindolol on the quality of sleep does not clearly explain the fact that heart rate did not drop during the night.

Renal haemodynamic parameters were not influenced by bopindolol treatment of human hypertensives.

Duration of action

In all animal and human studies the long duration of action of bopindolol is obvious. Bopindolol, being a prodrug, is hydrolysed rapidly after oral administration. Hydrolysed bopindolol (HBP) is the active metabolite, inducing β-blockade of long duration, and possesses a plasma half-life of approximately 4 h, which is far too short to explain the long duration of action. However, a linear relationship between the degree of induced β-receptor blockade and log plasma concentration of HBP can be demonstrated. The shallow slope of this relationship might be caused by long persistence of the drug at β-receptors in the cardiovascular system. Pharmacokinetic, though rather indirect arguments would not suggest a relevant role of an active metabolite with a long half-life. The 1 : 1 correlation between concentrations measured by radioreceptor assay and liquid chromatography would argue against the existence of such an active metabolite. However, this possibility is only rejected upon theoretical and indirect grounds and therefore remains worth investigation in a more direct manner.

The long duration of action of bopindolol was also demonstrated by the fact that the dosage of 8 mg once a week was shown to be effective in maintaining the blood pressure lowering achieved with a daily dose of 1–2 mg in hypertensive patients.

It remains unanswered whether administration once weekly would improve patient compliance or not, but this novel dosage schedule in antihypertensive treatment also appears worth further, more thorough investigation.

Side-effects and safety

Bopindolol should be expected to display the usual side-effect pattern of a $\beta_1 + \beta_2$ (non-selective) adrenoceptor antagonist. Indeed, unexpected side-effects have not been reported so far and the drug appears to be well tolerated. It may be expected to induce bronchoconstriction in patients with obstructive airways disease, but very few data on this subject are available at present.

In essential hypertensives appropriately treated with bopindolol, total cholesterol, low density lipoprotein (LDL)-cholesterol and high density lipoprotein (HDL)-cholesterol remained unchanged, whereas a slight but probably irrelevant increase in triglycerides was observed. The fact that HDL-cholesterol is not reduced might be favourable. The very modest effect of bopindolol on plasma lipids resembles that of β-blockers with ISA. The effect on lipid profile also resembles that of prazosin, but it is certainly not caused by the fall in blood pressure or by the blunting of sympathetic stimuli.

Also in studies on a larger scale, bopindolol appeared to be well tolerated and so far there are no clear indications that this new β-adrenoceptor antagonist caused cold hand and feet, a very frequently reported side-effect of all β-blockers developed to date. In a large scale study by Swiss general practitioners (see below) bopindolol even caused a few improvements, for instance a reduction of the incidence and severity of headache and the feeling of light-headedness. In hypertensive patients with a reduced left ventricular ejection fraction (LVEF) bopindolol treatment led to a satisfactory control of hypertension without any negative effect on LVEF. A similar profile was found for metoprolol.

The long duration of the therapeutic effect of bopindolol raises the question whether its adverse reactions would also persist for a concomitant long period. This problem remains to be investigated.

Efficacy of antihypertensive treatment

The efficacy of bopindolol in the treatment of mild to moderate essential hypertension has been established in several studies, including a large scale study by Swiss general practitioners. Both in monotherapy and when combined with a thiazide diuretic, bopindolol appeared an effective antihypertensive, with a responder rate in the order of magnitude of 70% of the patients treated. The efficacy of bopindolol was at least as high as that of metoprolol. Its antihypertensive efficacy was clearly independent of the patients' age, thus weakening the too easily accepted hypothesis that β-blockers should preferably be used in younger hypertensives and rather not in older patients. Also in a limited number of cases of severe hypertension bopindolol proved effective.

Adverse reactions were within the profile of β-adrenoceptor blockade and as a rule the drug was well tolerated. A few subjective improvements induced by bopindolol have already been discussed above.

Antianginal activity

In a limited number of patients ($n=10$) with stable angina, bopindolol once daily (1–4 mg by mouth) proved as effective as metoprolol twice daily in reducing the frequency and the severity of anginal attacks, accompanied by a reduced consumption of nitroglycerine. Side-effects of bopindolol were minor and clinically irrelevant.

Overall profile of bopindolol

In conclusion, the available data allows us to briefly characterize bopindolol by the following profile:

bopindolol, a very potent, non-selective $\beta_1+\beta_2$-adrenoceptor blocking agent is a pro-drug, with an extremely long duration of action. It displays a modest degree of ISA in certain models, but this property can hardly or inconsistently be demonstrated in human haemodynamic studies. Its long duration of action cannot be explained by plasma pharmacokinetics only. Long persistence at the receptor level or the formation of an active metabolite with a long half-life may cause the long duration of action, which allows once daily and possibly once weekly administration.

The drug is effective in mild and moderate hypertension and displays its efficacy independent of the patients' age. It is well tolerated and its side-effects remain within the pattern to be expected for non-selective β-blockers. Its lipid profile remains virtually neutral and does not appear as an additional coronary risk factor.

Preliminary data indicate its possible use as an antianginal drug.

Recommendations for further investigations: what remains to be done?

The participants of the round table conference would like to put forward the following suggestions concerning useful future investigations on bopindolol:

1. There are many interesting aspects of the pharmacology of bopindolol which could be investigated.
2. More work should be performed on biotransformation and elimination of HBP in humans. In particular one would like to know whether an active metabolite is formed with a possible long duration of action, possessing ISA or not. Renal elimination in humans should also be studied quantitatively.
3. Attempts to establish the role of presynaptic β_2-receptors in the antihypertensive effect would not only be useful for bopindolol, but for β-blockers in general.
4. It would be of great interest to develop a method allowing quantification of the degree of ISA in humans of bopindolol, HBP and of other β-blockers in general.
5. A better explanation of the long duration of the effect of bopindolol is required. Both the drug's persistence at the receptor level and the possibility of a long acting metabolite (see 1) should be investigated. This should include investigations of the receptor binding kinetics and of changes in the receptor population.
6. The possibility of once weekly administration of bopindolol and the implications of such a schedule for patient compliance in antihypertensive treatment should be investigated in more detail.
7. A dosage of 1–2 mg daily antihypertensive treatment appears to involve the upper part of the drug's dose response curve. For this reason it appears of interest to study the efficacy of doses lower than 1 mg.
8. In view of the drug's long duration of action the question whether side-effects are concomitantly persistent should be studied.
9. The influence of bopindolol on the quality of sleep should be studied, together with its affinity for serotonine (5HT)-receptors, since the latter receptors are probably involved in central nervous side-effects of β-blockers.

10. More data should be gathered concerning the interaction between bopindolol and other drugs.
11. Other indications than hypertension should be explored. Not only cardiological applications like angina pectoris, but other fields like migraine and glaucoma simplex would be worthwhile to study as potential therapeutic goals for bopindolol.